The Gay Science

T0386182

Since the onset of the HIV epidemic, the behaviour of men who have sex with men has been subject to intense scrutiny on the part of the behavioural and sociomedical sciences. What happens when we consider the work of these sciences to be not merely descriptive, but also constitutive of the realities it describes? *The Gay Science* pays attention to lived experiences of sex, drugs and the scientific practices that make these experiences intelligible. Through a series of empirically and historically detailed case studies, the book examines how new technologies and scientific artifacts – such as antiretroviral therapy, digital hookup apps and research methods – mediate sexual encounters and shape the worlds and self-practices of men who have sex with men.

Rather than debunking scientific practices or minimising their significance, *The Gay Science* approaches these practices as ways in which we 'learn to be affected' by HIV. It explores what knowledge practices best engage us, move us and increase our powers and capacities for action. The book includes an historical analysis of drug use as a significant element in the formation of urban gay cultures; constructivist accounts of the emergence of barebacking and chemsex; a performative response to Pre-Exposure Prophylaxis and its uptake; and, a speculative analysis of ways of thinking and doing sexual community in the digital context.

Combining insights from queer theory, process philosophy and science and technology studies to develop an original approach to the analysis of sexuality, drug use, public health and digital practices, this book demonstrates the ontological consequences of different modes of attending to risk and pleasure. It is suitable for those interested in cultural studies, sociology, gender and sexuality studies, digital culture, public health and drug and alcohol studies.

Kane Race is Associate Professor of Gender and Cultural Studies at the University of Sydney, Australia. He is the convenor of the Queer Contingent of Unharm and the author of *Pleasure Consuming Medicine: The Queer Politics of Drugs* (2009).

Sexuality, Culture and Health series

https://www.routledge.com/Sexuality-Culture-and-Health/book-series/SCH

Edited by Peter Aggleton, University of New South Wales, Australia
Richard Parker, Columbia University, New York, USA
Sonia Corrêa, ABIA, Rio de Janeiro, Brazil
Gary Dowsett, La Trobe University, Melbourne, Australia
Shirley Lindenbaum, City University of New York, USA

This series of books offers cutting-edge analysis, current theoretical perspectives and up-to-the-minute ideas concerning the interface between sexuality, public health, human rights, culture and social development. It adopts a global and interdisciplinary perspective in which the needs of poorer countries are given equal status to those of richer nations. Books are written with a broad range of readers in mind, and will be invaluable to students, academics and those working in policy and practice. The series also aims to serve as a spur to practical action in an increasingly globalised world.

Technologies of Sexuality, Identity and Sexual Health
Edited by Lenore Manderson

Understanding Global Sexualities: New Frontiers
Edited by Peter Aggleton, Paul Boyce, Henrietta L. Moore and Richard Parker

Men who Sell Sex: Global Perspectives
Edited by Peter Aggleton and Richard Parker

Sex and Sexualities in Contemporary Indonesia: Sexual Politics, Health, Diversity and Representations
Edited by Linda Rae Bennett and Sharyn Graham Davies

Culture, Health and Sexuality: An Introduction
Edited by Peter Aggleton and Richard Parker

The Gay Science: Intimate Experiments with the Problem of HIV
Kane Race

The Gay Science

Intimate Experiments with the Problem
of HIV

Kane Race

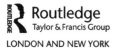
Routledge
Taylor & Francis Group

LONDON AND NEW YORK

First published 2018
by Routledge
2 Park Square, Milton Park, Abingdon, Oxon OX14 4RN

and by Routledge
711 Third Avenue, New York, NY 10017

First issued in paperback 2018

Routledge is an imprint of the Taylor & Francis Group, an informa business

© 2018 Kane Race

British Library Cataloguing-in-Publication Data
A catalogue record for this book is available from the British Library

Library of Congress Cataloging-in-Publication Data
Names: Race, Kane, author.
Title: Gay science: intimate experiments with the problem of HIV /
    Kane Race.
Description: Abingdon, Oxon; New York, NY: Routledge, 2018. |
    Series: Sexuality, culture and health series | Includes
    bibliographical references and index.
Identifiers: LCCN 2017014362| ISBN 9781138683822 (hardback) |
    ISBN 9781315544328 (ebook)
Subjects: LCSH: HIV infections—Australia—Prevention—Social
    aspects. | Gay men—Sexual behavior—Australia. | Gay men—
    Health risk assessment—Australia. | Health behavior—Australia.
Classification: LCC RA643.86.A8 R33 2018 | DDC
    614.5/99392086642—dc23LC record available at https://lccn.loc.
    gov/2017014362

ISBN 13: 978-1-138-31671-3 (pbk)
ISBN 13: 978-1-138-68382-2 (hbk)

Typeset in Garamond
by Swales & Willis Ltd, Exeter, Devon, UK

This book is dedicated to Susan Kippax, for teaching us how to enjoy the empirical.

"*The Gay Science* is a gift. Working across art, economics, epidemiology, sociology, ethnography and critical theories of personhood and sexuality, Kane Race freshens up how we see the medical and sexual chemistry of contemporary gayness. Drugs and new media, parties and apps create new lifeworlds for sex and intimacy–managing them and revising the event of intimate encounters. Philosophically engaged and fun to read, *The Gay Science* feels out for ways to phrase queer sexuality's current transitional phase". *Lauren Berlant, George M. Pullman Distinguished Service Professor, The University of Chicago, USA*

"In *The Gay Science*, Kane Race moves constantly, seamlessly, and elegantly back and forth between cutting-edge social theory and the new, intimate worlds of sex and drugs. His fine-tuned investigations of risks and pleasures reveal the intricate connections of biomedicine, criminal law, and new digital infrastructures in the forging of sexual practices and the regulation of sexual subjects. This fascinating and important book will ignite debate about the prospects for enacting what Race provocatively terms 'counterpublic health'." *Steven Epstein, Professor of Sociology and John C. Shaffer Professor in the Humanities, Northwestern University, USA*

Contents

Acknowledgements

This book began its life more than ten years ago when the topic of barebacking made me consider how to think about pleasure and risk. For his crucial interest, encouragement and guidance at that time I thank David Halperin, who helped me realise that I had things to discuss with people outside my world, that I was capable of doing so and that taking such a risk might actually be worthwhile. Special thanks also to Marsha Rosengarten and Gay Hawkins for their ongoing encouragement over the years, their extraordinary minds, the extensive feedback they have given me and the sustenance I have experienced in thinking with them.

I have learnt from many people while undertaking this work. I have particularly appreciated the contributions of Barry Adam, Kath Albury, Dennis Altman, Judith Auerbach, Ruth Barcan, Lauren Berlant, the late Alan Brotherton, Rebecca Brown, Jean Burgess, Gus Cairns, William Caroline, David Caron, Ross Chambers, Jerry Chang, the late June Crawford, Maital Dar, Rosalyn Diprose, Ben Drayton, Catherine Driscoll, Ross Duffin, Jeanne Ellard, Nadine Ezard, Suzanne Fraser, Laurent Gaissad, Laurindo Garcia, Moira Gatens, William Gaver, Davi Martinelli Gonçalves, Robert Grant, Monica Greco, Melissa Gregg, Antoine Hennion, Neville Hoad, Martin Holt, Geoff Honnor, Trevor Hoppe, Annamarie Jagose, Jess Kean, Helen Keane, Adrian Kerr, Paul Kidd, Kimberly Koester, Corey Knobel, Johann Kolstee, Declan Kuch, Kari Lancaster, Tess Lea, Cath Le Couteur, Julie Letts, Ben Light, Heather Love, Brent Mackie, Peta Malins, Gail Mason, Fiona McGregor, Viv McGregor, David McInnes, Suzie McLean, Mike Michael, Anne-Lise Middelthon, David Moore, Ed Moreno, Meaghan Morris, Dean Murphy, Darryl O'Donnell, Johnny Pappas, Jane Park, Amie Elizabeth Parry, Robert Payne, Nick Perret, Anne Pollock, Fiona Probyn-Rapsey, Vololona Rabeharisoa, Lionel Rabie, Alison Ritter, the late Eric Rofes, Martin Savransky, John Sinatore, Gavin Smith, Aldo Spina, Zahra Stardust, Niamh Stephenson, David Stuart, Steven Tomsen, Mathieu Trachman, Will Tregoning, kylie valentine, Catherine Waldby, Russell Westacott, Alex Wilkie and Richard Williamson.

I have also benefited a great deal from the opportunities I have had to share my thinking with unfamiliar audiences. For their engagement with this work I am especially grateful to Hans Tao-Ming Huang and his colleagues from the Center for the Study of Sexualities at National Central University Taiwan; Kåre Moen and friends from the Institute of Health & Society at the University of Oslo; Vincent Douris, Veronica Noseda and colleagues from Sidaction, Paris; Mark Davis from the School of Social Sciences at Monash University; Amy Dobson and Nicholas Carah and participants in the first *Digital Intimacies* conference at the University of Queensland; Ann Pellegrini and colleagues from the Center for the Study of Gender and Sexuality at New York University; Antoine Hennion and colleagues from the Centre de Sociologie de l'Innovation at MINES Paris Tech; my friends and colleagues at Goldsmith's Unit of Play and Interaction Research Studio; Melissa Gregg and colleagues from the Intel User Experience Lab; Robert Grant and colleagues from the Gladstone Institute and UCSF; Larissa Hjorth and colleagues from the Digital Ethnography Research Centre at RMIT University; Tamas Bereczky and colleagues from the European AIDS Treatment Group; my friends and colleagues from the Australian Federation of AIDS Organisations, the Australian Research Centre for Sex, Health & Society at La Trobe University and the Centre for Social Research in Health at the University of New South Wales; my comrades in the Unharm Queer Contingent; and my wonderful colleagues, students and teachers from the Department of Gender & Cultural Studies, University of Sydney, especially Elspeth Probyn, who knows a thing or two about affective climates and puts that know-how to work in ways that contribute greatly to an energising, warm and enjoyable departmental environment.

This book was made possible by a grant from the Australian Research Council Discovery Scheme, and I thank this funding body for supporting my project 'Changing Spaces of HIV Prevention: A Cultural Analysis of Transformations in Sexual Sociability Among Gay and Homosexually Active Men' (DP120101990). Thanks to Dion Kagan for his sterling research assistance, as well as his patience and enthusiasm for my ideas. Many thanks to the gay men we interviewed for this project for sharing their time and insights. I am most grateful to Peter Aggleton for taking an interest in my work and for his very helpful advice, encouragement, support and feedback over the years, especially during the final stages of this work, which made pulling this book together much easier than it might otherwise have been. Thanks also to Grace McInnes and the editorial team at Routledge for their patience, professionalism and flexibility.

This book reworks arguments from a number of my previously published articles and book chapters. I thank the publishers for permission to reproduce sections from:

Race, K. 2007. Engaging in a culture of barebacking: Gay men and the risk of HIV prevention. In K. Hannah-Moffatt & P. O'Malley (eds.) *Gendered Risks*. Oxon: Routledge-Cavendish, pp. 99–126.

Race, K. 2010. Click here for HIV status: Shifting templates of sexual negotiation. *Emotion, Space and Society*, 3(1), pp. 7–14.

Race, K., 2011. Party animals: The significance of drug practices in the materialization of urban gay identity. In S. Fraser & D. Moore (eds.) *The Drug Effect*. Melbourne: Cambridge University Press, pp. 35–56.

Race, K. 2012. Framing responsibility: HIV, biomedical prevention, and the performativity of the law. *Journal of Bioethical Inquiry*, 9(3), pp. 327–338.

Race, K., 2015. 'Party and play': Online hook-up devices and the emergence of PNP practices among gay men. *Sexualities*, 18(3), pp. 253–275.

Race, K. 2015. Speculative pragmatism and intimate arrangements: Online hook-up devices in gay life. *Culture, Health & Sexuality*, 17(4), pp. 496–511.

Race, K. 2016. Reluctant objects: Sexual pleasure as a problem for HIV biomedical prevention. *GLQ: A Journal of Lesbian and Gay Studies*, 22(1), pp. 1–31.

This book would never have been possible were it not for the extraordinary contribution that Susan Kippax has made to HIV prevention. Thank you, Sue, for your energy, support and agitation over many years – I hope you enjoy this book. Naturally, I must thank my mother and father for bearing me: I look forward to a time when *The Gay Science* is as easy to live with as *Plastic Water*. Finally, I can't imagine finishing this work in quite the way I have were it not for my unexpected encounter with Stephan Omeros, beautiful stranger, whose consistent affection, patience, generosity, idiocy and good humour has taught me so much about gay life, pleasure and what it means to love another. For this and more, I'm eternally grateful.

Kane Race
Sydney, 28 February 2017

What if some day or night a demon were to steal into your loneliest loneliness and say to you, 'This life as you now live it and have lived it you will have to live once again and innumerable times again; and there will be nothing new in it, but every pain and every joy and every thought and sigh and everything unbearably small or great in your life must return to you. . . . Would you not throw yourself down and gnash your teeth and curse the demon who spoke thus? Or have you once experienced a tremendous moment when you would have answered him: 'You are a god, and never have I heard anything more divine'?

(Nietzsche, *The Gay Science*, 2001, p. 194 [orig. 1882])

1 The gay science

Intimate experiments with the problem of HIV

Hedonia:	Drink this.
Dale Arden:	What is it?
Hedonia:	It has no name. Many brave men died to bring it here from the Galaxy of Pleasure . . .
Dale Arden:	Will it make me forget?
Hedonia:	No, but it will make you not mind remembering

(Flash Gordon, 1980, dir. M. Hodges)

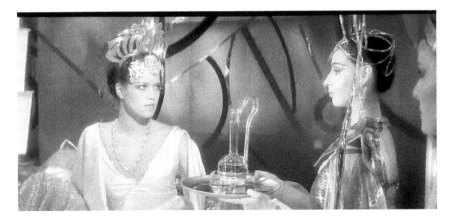

Figure 1.1 Hedonia's potion.

Still from *Flash Gordon*, 1980. Courtesy of the Dino De Laurentiis Company

Every effort has been made to contact copyright-holders. Please advise the publisher of any errors or omissions, and these will be corrected in subsequent editions.

The demon of Nietzsche's *Gay Science* (2001, p. 194) steals into our loneliest loneliness with a speculative riddle that asks us what we might make of our lives were every moment to be repeated *ad infinitum*. The demon's thought-experiment sparks a question that is daunting, ethical, practical and entirely worldly in its implications: what manner of relating to the events of the present might we devise that would enable us to bear the possibility of their infinite recurrence? This is an active and open question, and one that deserves many responses. But when it comes to the prospect of unbearable or unwanted sex, Universal Pictures' *Flash Gordon* (Hodges 1980) proposes a partial antidote: a strange potion brought by brave men from the Galaxy of Pleasure, whose arduous voyage is said to have cost many of them their lives. The concubine Hedonia advises that the potion won't knock you out or erase the dreaded experience so much as *mediate* it so that the prospect of remembering it will not seem so bad. Read alongside and against each other, these quivering scenes of anticipation and apprehension prefigure many of the questions and topics this book addresses. How should we engage a world that is at risk of closing in on people or completely shutting down, all because of the seemingly unbearable dangers, risks and apprehensions that persistently pervade sex even in the fourth decade of the HIV epidemic? What are the risks and benefits of different ways of apprehending and mediating sexual and other risky experiences? These questions require individual responses, but they also constitute practical, technical and public matters of concern: how should *we* (as people at risk, scientists, policy-makers, affected communities, sexual subjects and social actors) grasp the HIV epidemic and the relations through which the virus is transmitted? No one could ever hope to answer such questions once and for all. Instead, this book ventures a partial response to such matters in the hope of generating new interest in the question of how we might best attend to such problems and multiply our collective capacities for responsiveness.

This book is about the *risks* and *pleasures* of HIV science – its involvement in the production of situations it cannot anticipate, its capacity to reorganise social and material worlds. I investigate the encounter between HIV social science and the sexual practices of gay and other men who have sex with men in the urban centres of Australia over the past two decades with reference to comparable developments in Europe, the USA and Canada. Commonly regarded as birthplaces of modern gay identity, these locations persist as key sites of HIV prevalence among gay and other men who have sex with men (MSM). But they have also given rise to distinctive innovations in HIV prevention, education, research and care. Scientific conceptions of sexual risk have been transformed in their encounter with this population, just as this group's sexual practices have been transformed in its encounter with HIV science. This book analyses some of the ways this has taken place to affirm the transformative potential of both science and sex.

Since the beginning of the epidemic, the behaviour of MSM has been subject to intense scrutiny on the part of the sociomedical sciences. But here

I will approach this as more than just another instance of pervasive social control and surveillance. Certainly, the HIV policy field has relied upon the disciplinary practices of the human sciences in its efforts to control the spread of the epidemic. But these sciences are also among the principal ways in which those at risk *learn to be affected* by HIV. This raises a question whose significance I take to be no less critical than it is practical: what knowledge practices might best engage the relevant publics, move them and increase their powers and capacities for action?

As a gay man who started working in HIV social research in 1997 – the year the effectiveness of combination therapy was announced to the world – I do not claim to stand outside this history as some sort of detached or neutral observer. These events have transformed me in ways I couldn't have anticipated at that time. I was diagnosed as HIV positive the year before. Whether I like it or not, this book will demonstrate some of the implications of the emotional and social situation of the researcher for the research process. The field of cultural studies has spent much time and effort reckoning with the risks and benefits of 'acknowledging partiality and admitting one's attraction to the culture under investigation' (Gregg 2006, p. 142). But in this statement culture appears external to the subject investigating it. More often than not, I have found myself in the midst of things. Acknowledging one's social and emotional location and how it shapes one's research is beset with difficulties, but in this book I affirm the necessity of trying to do so. In this sense, this book can be situated as an exercise in cultural studies of science and sexuality: it presents a series of personal and social experiments with the problem of HIV.

Gay science

My title pays homage to 'The Gay Science', an interview with Michel Foucault that Jean Bitoux conducted in 1978, which also happened to be one of the first occasions Foucault discussed his homosexuality publicly (Foucault 2011; Halperin 2011). The interview sheds light on the sort of intervention Foucault hoped to make in the first volume of *The History of Sexuality* (1984), the publication of which had met with confusion and perplexity on the part of sexual liberationists in France. Rather than trying to undermine activist efforts, Foucault insisted in this interview that his entrée into the history of sexuality was intended to effect a 'change in the axis' of the sexual liberation movements (2011, p. 388). In place of 'sex-desire', he had argued that 'bodies and pleasures' – 'in their multiplicity and their possibility of resistance' – ought to form the rallying point against the regime of sexuality (Foucault 1984, p. 157). But what is the difference between 'sex-desire' and 'bodies and pleasures'? In 'The Gay Science', Foucault explained his view that the liberationist enthusiasm for uncovering and liberating the truth of desire was likely to lead right back into the clutches of therapeutic power. Given the medical and psychological stranglehold on the theorisation of desire, the concept was all too prone to operate as:

a kind of instrument for establishing the intelligibility of a sexual pleasure and thus for standardizing it in terms of normality. Tell me what your desire is, and I'll tell you who you are. I'll tell you if you're sick or not.

(2011, p. 389)

To counter this situation, Foucault conceives pleasure in the following terms:

[B]y using the word pleasure, which in the end means nothing, which is still, it seems to me, rather empty of content and unsullied by possible uses – in treating pleasure ultimately as nothing other than an event, an event that happens, that happens, I would say, outside the subject, or at the limit of the subject, or between two subjects, in this something that is neither of the body nor of the soul, neither outside nor inside – don't we have here, in trying to reflect a bit on this notion of pleasure, a means of avoiding the entire psychological and medical armature that was built into the traditional notion of desire?

(2011, pp. 389–90)

The Gay Science takes inspiration from the idea of pleasure as an event, and uses it to propose a novel way of grasping the world-changing effects not only of pleasure, but also science and the government of risk. To do this, I draw from work in the fields of science and technology studies and the philosophy of science, where the concept of the event has been used to displace the sovereign assurance implicit in the notion of the scientific 'discoverer' (Whitehead & Sherburne 1981; Latour 1999; Stengers 2000; Fraser 2010; Michael 2012). An event directs attention to the transformations undergone by all the elements that enter into it, including the figure of the scientist or the human subject. In treating pleasure and science as similarly involved in processes of eventuation, I hope to engender more active forms of attention to the manner in which their constituent elements come together, their contingencies and the differences these make to worlds and lives.

Foucault's distinction between pleasure and desire can be understood as a sophisticated intervention into given arrangements of knowledge and power and the disciplinary operation of the human sciences. It tackles conventional assumptions about who should get to define erotic experience and make authoritative determinations about individuals on this basis (i.e. medical experts or the subjects in question?). Promoting 'the claims of bodies, pleasures and knowledges, in their multiplicity and their possibility of resistance' requires at least some degree of interest and engagement with the situations, attachments and trajectories of particular bodies and more: it constitutes these bodies as sources of expertise and political/pragmatic possibility (Foucault 1984, p. 157). The tradition of HIV social science that informs much of my work in this field has focused on the social pragmatics of pleasure rather than the psychology of desire. I believe Foucault's distinction between desire and pleasure provides a basis for differentiating between different modes of sexuality and drug research and assessing their disciplinary implications (Race 2008). Rather than pathologising desires to typecast and administer individuals, this book promotes a more pragmatic, situated and speculative approach to the experience of bodies and pleasures with the aim of staving off some of the more deterministic effects of both the behavioural sciences and identity politics.

The title of Bitoux's interview pays homage, in turn, to Nietzsche's philosophical work *The Gay Science* (2001), a book of poems and aphorisms whose key provocation is that science has never been about truth but is rightly grounded in the passions of the body – 'the passion of the knowledge seeker is a very erotic drive', as Babich puts it (2006, p. 102). Nietzsche's *Gay Science* expresses an opposition to the nineteenth-century ideals of a positivist, measuring science that many modern empiricists may find alarming. It is nonetheless dedicated to the notion of science as a practice of fearless questioning; thus the question of method becomes a central problem. Nietzsche hoped to devise an affirmative style of thought that could make sense of painful experiences of the body – illness, suffering, disappointment, misrecognition and death – to enact a transmutation of shame in the activity of thought. 'To what extent can truth endure incorporation?' Nietzsche asks. 'That is the question, that is the experiment' (2001, p. 112) – a pertinent question for HIV prevention, if ever there was one.

'A "gay" science, emphasizing light and laughter, has well-known risks', Babich observes, for 'success in the parodic art of laughter seems to block the seriousness of science' (2006, p. 97). Indeed, Nietzsche's contemporaries balked at his project: '"Gay" it may be, but it is certainly not "science"', they reportedly objected (cited in Babich 2006, p. 97). But those who dismiss the applicability of Nietzsche's argument to the practices of modern science may be writing his work off a little too hastily. *The Gay Science* conceived science as both an ascetic and empirical practice to promote the profoundly serious endeavour of playing or experimenting with yourself in your own thinking, 'varying the effects of health, illness, convalescence, or the persistence of illness and pain on thought itself', as Babich puts it (2006, p. 99). Rather than denying bodily experience, Nietzsche promotes an approach to knowledge that would acknowledge and affirm such experiences. 'Something as fundamental as our erotic attachment to life . . . is at issue' in this work (Pippin 2000, p. 142).

Problems as intimate experiments

The connections between the passionate science promoted by Nietzsche and Foucault's project in *The History of Sexuality* have yet to be explored in sufficient detail, but one key to these connections might be found in Foucault's concept of *problematisation*. Foucault first deployed the concept to refer to the 'ensemble of discursive and nondiscursive practices that make something enter into the play of true and false and constitute it as an object of thought' (cited in Rabinow 2005, p. 43). As an analytic approach, the term is most familiar among governmentality scholars, who take the analysis of problematisations to enable a 'freeing up' of possibilities, since it allows one to imagine how a given problem-situation might be otherwise enacted on the basis of a different set of perceptions, framings and practices (Rabinow 2005, p. 43). Many of the chapters in this book draw on this approach to wrestle with given ways of understanding certain problems in the field of HIV and make proposals about how they might be formulated or enacted otherwise. However, problematisation remains a rather disembodied affair within much of the governmentality scholarship, and this aspect obstructs exploration of some of the more radical implications of this approach. It is striking that Foucault elaborates his understanding of problematisation towards the end of his life, in the midst of undertaking genealogical research on the history of sexuality, for example. From the opening pages of *The Use of Pleasure*, the second volume of *The History of Sexuality*, it is clear Foucault regards this 'exercise of oneself in the activity of thought' as a form of ascesis in terms that resonate with Nietzsche's emphasis on playing or experimenting with the body (1990, p. 9). In his introduction to the volume, Foucault asks, 'what would be the value of the passion for knowledge if it resulted only in a certain amount of knowledgeableness, and not, in one way or another . . . in the knower's straying afield of himself?' (1990, p. 8). The emphasis here on *straying afield of* the self suggests an approach to knowledge and research grounded in experiences of curiosity and pleasure, motivated by the need to think and feel otherwise. This emphasis recalls Foucault's remarks in a number of late interviews about the creative possibilities of sex, drugs and pleasure which he illustrated with reference to the experimental cultures of gay life he encountered in the late 1970s (Foucault 1997a, 1997b, 2011). In these interviews, Foucault discusses the possibilities of self-overcoming through experimenting with bodies and pleasures and the possibility this holds of constructing new modes of self-relation – relations of 'differentiation, of creation, of innovation' rather than self-same identity (1997a, p. 166).

While writing this book I had the opportunity to visit Auguste Rodin's 1901 sculpture *The Thinker* – 'in the flesh', as it were. Looming over the gardens of the Musée Rodin – just a stone's throw from the Dôme des Invalides – *The Thinker* dramatically demonstrates the participation of the body in the activity of thought. Rodin wrote about his sculpture:

> What makes my Thinker think is that he thinks not only with his brain, with his knitted brow, his distended nostrils and compressed lips, but with every muscle of his arms, back and legs, with his clenched fist and gripping toes.
>
> (National Gallery of Art 2016)

The statement departs significantly from the presuppositions of Cartesian dualism: Rodin's *Thinker* powerfully demonstrates the embodied processes 'through which being offers itself to be, necessarily, thought – and the practices on the basis of which these problematizations were formed' (Foucault 1990, p. 11).

Problematisation is such an unwieldy term: I think problem should be a verb. The word draws its origins from the Greek word πρόβλημα (próblēma), which means to throw forth or propose. As scholars as diverse as Iris Marion Young (1980) and Marcel Mauss (1973) have shown, throwing is a technique of the body: there are *ways of throwing*. This invites us to conceive of problems as performative actions, embodied gestures; practical wagers on the world – ways of doing things that can be experimented with and transformed. The form they take stems from particular manners of relating to the world – embodied habits and apprehensions – that are themselves keenly attuned to particular objectives and concerns. While Foucault was careful to emphasise that there are constraints at work in any given process of problematisation, he also argued there are always several possible ways of responding to 'the same ensemble of difficulties' – of making any given ensemble of difficulties into 'problems to which diverse solutions are proposed' (Rabinow 2005, p. 43). Conceiving *probleming* as a way of throwing forth, an enacted gesture, might enable a better appreciation of the connections between bodily experiments and transformative thought.

Experiments with bodies and pleasures have also featured prominently – indeed notoriously – in urban gay subcultures both historically and currently. Experimentation with sex, drugs and intimate relations constitutes the central focus of several chapters of this book. But rather than read these activities as signs of pathology and/or disorder, I approach them as attempts to reconfigure the terms of experience: exercises of the self in the activity of feeling and/or thought. These experimental activities can be approached as attempts to change some of the problems that have confronted queer lives historically. They have produced transformations in the ways people experience and practise pleasure, the ways we experience our bodily capacities and work on them, the ways we relate to each other and feel the world and more. Such practices are no less prevalent or relevant today as we enter the fourth decade of HIV. Not only have these experiments served as situated attempts to 'produce transformations' (more or less successfully, in different instances):[1] they have changed the way we think, research and govern ourselves and others in the time of HIV. Generative of – and set in motion by – new forms of agency and *probleming*, this book situates these activities as intimate experiments with the problem of HIV.

Gay, all too gay

Some readers might criticise this book's focus on 'gay and other men who have sex with men' – a category that HIV discourse has made into a particular sort of epistemic object, as one of its 'Key Affected Populations'. And certainly, this is one limitation of the approach I adopt – the locus of the intimate experiments undertaken in this work. But this population is all too prone to being conceived as a more or less homogenous group with its own sexual and cultural dynamics that neatly distinguish it from other populations affected by HIV. While such distinctions are sociologically and anthropologically justified to some extent (gay lives in Sydney or London are radically different to the lives of Sub-Saharan women and girls, or the conditions faced by injecting drug-users in Eastern Europe in their everyday lives), the imputed homogeneity of this category can override considerations of how the abstractions of race, class, location, gender and transgender identity cut across and create differences for and within gay life.

Conscious of such objections, I suggest the term 'gay' need not refer to the fixed, stable or homogenous identity it is often presumed or imagined to be. Even when supplemented with the apparently ahistorical descriptor 'men who have sex with men', the category 'gay men' inevitably fails to capture or reflect the heterogeneous, evolving and overlapping constituencies it tries to name. Not only was the 'gay community' that first mobilised in response to HIV crucially informed by the women's health and civil rights movements; it was generously frequented by lesbians, cis-women, sex workers, people of colour and trans and gender diverse folk, who contributed to its social, cultural and political innovations and expressivity in crucial ways. Moreover, however enduringly the category persists as an administrative object, 'gay men' are not what they used to be. Over the past two decades, gay male identities have been radically and irrevocably transformed in their encounter with the biomedical, digital, technological and historical developments which this book conceives as the changing infrastructures of sexual life.

Given queer theory's well-trodden critique of the fixations of identity, the title of this book, *The Gay Science*, could only refer to some coherent, positivistic science of 'the gays' through some (particularly flippant) sleight of hand. Scholars of queer theory are rigorously trained these days to cite the exclusionary and regulatory effects of identity as just cause for its vigorous deconstruction, debunking and critical displacement. This book adopts a different approach to identity and its abstraction, inspired by the constructivism of philosophers of science such as Isabelle Stengers and A. N. Whitehead. This entails affirming the term gay in its constructed facticity as a governmental and scientific object (and social identity) – a real force in the world that shapes and constrains how we think about and organise responses to HIV. By slowing down and acknowledging the historicity of this category, I hope to reorient the work this term does, not by debunking it but by taking the problems it has emerged to address seriously. My aim here is to create new modes of thought and action that reformulate the problem that this term has come to assemble (see Halewood 2011, p. 59; Stengers 2008, pp. 101–2). The term might function as more than a descriptor of identity to describe a stance, or particular manner of relating to the world. Certainly, the encounter between HIV science and gay sex over the past two decades constitutes the substantive focus of this work, and my empirical investigations take sexual relations between men as their central focus (an emphasis for which I make no apology). But alongside their empirical insights, the case studies that together make up this book aim to demonstrate a mode of inquiry that I hope will promote more expansive and generative approaches to sex, health, risk and pleasure – what I am calling a gay science. I want to devise a set of stylistic and methodological practices that might be adapted by other researchers, thinkers and activists in relation to the problems that concern them.

By tweaking the term gay in this way so that it operates impersonally to characterise an approach to knowledge-creation (and not merely a descriptor of fixed identities), my purpose is certainly not to evacuate the term of its deep entanglement with homosexual history and politics. In an era characterised by the steady biomedicalisation of sexual experience, my use of the term is critically informed by its historic use on the part of gay liberationists to shake off the pathologising associations of homosexuality as a diagnostic category. Insofar as the term gay enabled activists to transpose homosexuality from its historical associations with abject shame and sickness into a source of joyful identification and pride, it instantiated precisely the sort of manoeuvre I wish to effect in relation to the pathologised cultures that populate present discourses of HIV prevention. Of course, the re-signification of homosexuality that use of the term *gay* has historically effectuated depends on its much longer chain of well-known etymological associations: reference texts list joyful, merry, happy, pleasant, light-hearted, delightful and delighted as among the historical meanings of the word. In this book I associate this series of joyful affects with a certain practical orientation to the world: one that takes delight in the unexpected; that finds a certain pleasure in buoyancy, contingency and movement; that attunes itself to the world's lively and eventful nature; that wonders at and allows itself to be altered by its chance encounters, surprises and paradoxes. This practical orientation operates as more than a personal philosophy for me: my hope with this work is that it will be freed up to operate more impersonally as a research ethic that can be adopted and adapted by others to change the terms of the problems that concern them and help realise possibilities that would otherwise be stifled or overlooked by the disciplinary practices that authorise their work.

A commitment to delight and buoyancy may irk readers invested in principles of queer negativity, or the critical figure of the killjoy, the political efficacy of which has been proposed in recent queer, feminist and anti-racist critique (Caserio et al. 2006; Ahmed 2010a). Far from disputing the achievements of these critical orientations, I will merely suggest that the affective open-ness I describe as gay is entirely consistent with the 'hap' of happiness – the pleasures of contingency that Sara Ahmed proposes as a radical rejoinder to the forms of happiness prescribed within regimes of reproductive futurity (Ahmed 2010b). Meanwhile, those whose lives have been irrevocably devastated by the ravages of HIV and AIDS may rankle at my invocation of joyful affects in proximity to a scene so steeped in precarity, loss, death, grief, exclusion, stigma, violence, neglect and repudiations of difference. On this point, it is worth remembering that the gleeful etymology I cited earlier finds its morbid counterpart in an equally sedimented set of historical associations. As early as the fourteenth century, alongside joy and delight, we find slurs such as lewd, lascivious, wanton, promiscuous, tramp, immoral, loafer, prostitute and vagabond as alternative meanings for the term gay. Evidently, the sense of contingency and surprise that furnishes gayness with so many of its affirmative possibilities is just as likely to provoke dread, contempt, abjection and recrimination.

Foucault's proposal I mentioned earlier to treat pleasure as an event can be read as an affirmation of the critical value of indeterminacy. Here, I take an event to be a transformative situation that somehow changes all those who participate in it in ways that none could have predicted precisely before entering into it.[2] As I suggested earlier, this concept can be used to make sense of scientific activity,[3] just as it can be used to characterise pleasure. In doing so, we might attend more carefully to their contingencies and the differences these make to worlds and lives. The manner in which HIV social research has been practised in Australia might serve as a case in point here: as a science, it has allowed itself to be transformed through its encounter with its objects. In what follows, I characterise the tradition of HIV social research that informs my work as a *gay science*: a science that seeks out the unexpected, that takes an interest in contingencies, that allows itself to be transformed by the surprises it encounters and strives to realise the creative possibilities they generate in the process.

The difference practice makes

How articulate is it possible to be about sexual practice? The question is the sort that triggers a million others. So let's rephrase it: how might sexual practice best be articulated in the interests of HIV prevention? Still we run up against a series of troubling presumptions: that talking about sex will redeem it; that it is possible to 'know' sex finally; that talking about it will help us work out *who we are* – the very presumptions Foucault warned us of in *The History of Sexuality* (1984). Foucault was conscious of the ways in which talk about sex can be used to classify and rank individuals:

> [t]ell me what your desire is, and I'll tell you who you are. I'll tell you if you're sick or not, I'll tell you if you're normal or not, and thus I'll be able to disqualify your desire or on the contrary requalify it.
>
> (Foucault 2011, p. 389)

Foucault argued that this is a regulatory procedure that attaches individuals to a particular social order; a social hierarchy that values normality above all other values and for this reason is deeply implicated in the production and maintenance of normativity and deviance. If one accepts the collective wisdom that stigmatising identities creates problems for HIV prevention, then talk about sex starts to seem like a very bad idea indeed.

But there is another sense of the word articulation that may help us dodge this regulatory game of identification and control and that places less emphasis on the 'truths' gleaned from confessional speech. This is the sense of the word given to us within science studies by Bruno Latour (1999, 2004a), for whom articulation does not describe the duty of subjects to speak their inner truths, but rather the responsibility of science to set itself up and arrange its procedures to allow for change and difference. Latour is concerned here with the making of scientific knowledge and, in particular, what it might take to produce 'good' articulations – by which he means *interesting* ones that move us and increase our powers and capacities for action (2004a). This is an argument about apparatuses of knowledge, the techniques and procedures that make data available to us; he wants to draw attention to the social and material settings in which particular apprehensions become possible. Here, articulation describes the quite material way in which one thing is connected to another. Think of the way in which various elements can be joined or fitted together to generate new connections and material capacities, and not just words and speech. In a richly articulated world, 'the more differences and mediations [we] become sensible to . . . the more *sensorium*, the more bodies, the more affections, the more realities will be registered' (Latour 2004a, pp. 212–13).

The difference between this conception and the regime of knowledge Foucault worried about is that the former does not set out to fix its objects or pin them down as though finally. Indeed, Latour's aim in this essay is to offer a set of ethical criteria for scientific practice, which he does by characterising 'good science' as that which gives its objects occasions to differ. But what does he mean by this? On his account, good science requires 'a passionately interested scientist who provides his or her object of study with as many occasions to show interest and to counter his or her questioning through the use of *its* own categories' (2004a, p. 218). In other words, it requires researchers to be prepared to put themselves at risk by asking the following, which is to affirm science as a transformative ascesis:

> Am I asking you the right questions? Have I devised the laboratory setting that allows me to change as fast as possible the questions I ask depending on the resistance of your behaviour to my questioning? Have I become sensitive to the possibility of your reacting to artifacts instead of my questions?
>
> (2004a, p. 216)

To policy-makers, these may seem like odd criteria for assessing scientific claims since the main requirement of science seems to be that it corresponds to the world 'out there' *as it really is* and accurately establishes and conveys 'the facts'. Yet these criteria are drawn from close engagement with the practices and values of scientists themselves, for whom an important question is not merely, 'is it scientific?' but also, '*is it interesting?*' (2004a, p. 215, emphasis added). Latour draws on the work of Isabelle Stengers and Vinciane Despret to arrive at these conclusions – philosophers of science who also happen to have worked as natural scientists. As a field of social inquiry, science studies emerged from close ethnographic observation of what it is that scientists actually *do*. Its approach to scientific practice conveys a world in process; a world made through the activity of a whole range of actors, including (but not limited to) scientists. In this body of work, scientists are depicted as not simply describing the world but participating in its making through their analytic practices. The significance of Latour's analysis is that it acknowledges the contribution of science to the making and transformation of the world while finding in 'good science' a spirit of humility. In acknowledging the agency of objects, by giving them occasions to differ, good science relinquishes the privilege of always being in command.

These criteria can be used to conceive some of the articulations of Australian HIV social science, which I first encountered and began to investigate as a researcher employed by the former National Centre in HIV Social Research (NCHSR) in Australia from 1997–2007. I joined the centre as a humanities graduate with an interest in cultural analysis of HIV but little experience of empirical social science. I may as well come clean and say I spent my first few years in the HIV sector wandering around scientific conferences wondering what on earth was going on. The genres and practices of HIV science (behavioural, epidemiological and biomedical) seemed to have an organising logic that was completely unfamiliar to me, trained as I was in humanities research. Faced with the prospect of having to participate in the bizarre rituals of this exotic planet, I quickly surmised that the only way to survive would be to adopt something like an ethnographic relation to the practices of the field. I gradually became familiar with the organising logics of HIV science and policy, while remaining keenly conscious of the forms of analysis and argumentation its formats habitually exclude (forms in which I happened to have been trained). This makes the Latourian frame I am invoking here particularly conducive for my purposes – to theorise some of the practices, methods, objects and affects of HIV social science. My aim, however, is not to debunk these practices or minimise their significance. As I mentioned earlier, I regard them as some of the principal ways in which communities affected by HIV 'learn to be affected, meaning "effectuated", moved, put into motion by other entities, humans or non-humans' (Latour 2004a, p. 205) – in this case, the realities of HIV.

The risk of practice

If there has been something distinctive about the articulations of HIV social science in Australia, this can largely be attributed to how it has conceived its object of research. This matter should be given 'careful consideration' according to Susan Kippax and Niamh Stephenson, who propose 'the object of study is *sexual practice* as opposed to sexual behaviour. This distinction is crucial' (2005, p. 362, emphasis added). And crucial it has been. But what is the difference between sexual behaviour and sexual practice? What is it that makes this distinction so pivotal? Behaviour is something that scientists believe they can extract from contexts, isolate, objectively measure and fix in individuals. By contrast, 'the object under consideration – sexual practice and its change – is fluid, embedded in specific social formations, and involves the negotiation of meaning' (2005, p. 361). It is embedded in particular historical situations, relations and formations. Its meanings and shape derive from these contexts. And it changes.

This is a fair enough definition of sexual activity that reflects certain disciplinary and theoretical commitments.[4] Particularly significant, though, is what this definition *does*, at the level of knowledge practice. Kippax and Stephenson draw out some of the relevant implications: 'Because social practice, the object being studied, is always situated in the everyday lives of those engaged in these practices, good evaluations work with and harness the meanings attributed to practice from the perspective of those involved' (2005, p. 367). In other words, this definition of sex interrupts any easy objectification of those it studies. It makes it very difficult to craft good knowledge about sex without some sort of practical input on their (which is often also to say our) part. In defining sex as a meaningful and variable activity, scientists put themselves at risk – the risk of never being able to assume that they know, once and for all or finally, what is going on in the sexual worlds they analyse. The ontological claim about 'what sex is' begins to unfold into a series of practical relations: conversations, exchanges, disputes, ruminations, interactions, contextualisations. It is as though the claim itself anticipates and suggests the performance of a more vigorous set of relations between the subjects and objects of scientific knowledge. And this is a symmetrical process: questions are raised, not only about how sex is done, but also about how science is done, or should be done – for example, whether it is using the right measures or asking the right questions of its field of study. In this sense, the concept of practice might be understood as putting science at risk in interesting and constructive ways. This definition of sexual practice promoted a particular set of relations between social research and those who participated in the sexual and risk cultures they studied, sometimes referred to in Australia as the 'partnership approach'. Whatever we decide to call this approach to sexuality research, the willingness to take these risks gave rise to some very significant insights.

Negotiated safety

In the context of the early AIDS crisis, gay communities invented an ethic of 'a condom every time', which was later taken up and promoted widely by professional health educators (Escoffier 1998; Race 2003). The condom code aimed to prevent HIV transmission between serodiscordant partners. By the early 1990s, certain changes in it were becoming apparent. Negotiated safety is a term coined to describe agreements made among regular, non-monogamous partners of HIV-negative status to dispense with condoms in the context of their primary relationship but maintain condom use in the context of sex that happens outside that relationship. When I joined the NCHSR in 1997, the centre was at the tail end of a process that distinguished Australian HIV social research from many of its international equivalents. Its researchers first articulated this practice in 1993 and, in the face of considerable resistance, maintained that it could be an effective strategy (Kippax et al. 1993). While other HIV scientists constructed the unprotected sex that was happening in similar contexts as 'relapse', this research team paid more attention to the contextual aspects of this practice and took the risk of constituting their study participants as agents. In other words, they were prepared to accept that the standard measure of risk practice (unprotected anal intercourse) might be questioned and countered by the categories, understandings and practices of those whom they were studying. What emerged from this process was a picture of gay men using multiple strategies to keep themselves safe, including strategies that had not yet been officially recognised.

It is difficult to fathom the professional bravery that the announcement of these findings involved. At the height of a devastating and frightening epidemic, the investment in safe sex norms was immense. Where NCHSR researchers saw 'negotiated safety', many US HIV specialists saw 'negotiated danger' (Ekstrand at al. 1993). But NCHSR researchers committed themselves to working with community educators to acknowledge what was going on and provide guidelines to make this practice safer (Kippax & Kinder 2002). Identifying this strategy involved a willingness to see past the sexual proprieties that emphasise the exclusivity of the long-term couple. It involved attuning science to the categories according to which research subjects were organising their sex lives. Many of the relevant practices were invisible from a conventional epidemiological perspective, which measured safety in terms of condom use only. Because epidemiology only counts *behaviours* such as unprotected sex, it was not well equipped to identify such *practices* as negotiated safety, since it makes little effort to determine the context in which sex occurs and the understandings surrounding it on the part of sexual actors. In this regard, the proposal of negotiated safety on the part of NCHSR researchers was better articulated with the everyday practices and self-understandings of those at risk than anything offered by standard epidemiological analyses of the situation.

The willingness of NCHSR researchers to draw on gay men's framing of their intimate practices to question the self-evidence of established categories of HIV prevention was all the more remarkable for the risks it took and the courageous attitude it embodied. By all accounts, when the claim was first made at an international conference that unprotected sex among gay men was not necessarily unsafe sex, you could have heard a pin drop. Effectively, these researchers were affirming a wider, more creative sense of agency on the part of those they studied as the latter negotiated the practical parameters of risk and safety and incorporated these parameters into their sex lives.

Evidence and articulation

There are two things about the articulation of negotiated safety that are worth expanding upon for the insight they give into some of the conditions in which these innovations took place, and for what they tell us about what it takes to participate as social scientists in a dynamic, constantly evolving field of every-day, intimate, sociomaterial experimentation. The first is that this proposition emerged from the careful analysis of robust quantitative data. In the social sciences, critiques of positivism abound, and the fact that governmental players only listen to 'the numbers' is a familiar lament. But in the organised fields of HIV prevention and drug policy, the numbers play a very important role. As well as guiding policy, it is often necessary to appeal to 'the evidence' to offset the political conservatism and reactionary moralism that always threat-ens to overwhelm pragmatic and rational public health initiatives. NCHSR researchers were always steadfast in their affirmation of the need for policy debate to be informed by evidence. Recognising how 'the numbers' matter in the policy field, their quantitative research team operated persuasively and rigorously in these terms. And yet the way the centre positioned its research and talked about its work undercut the tendency to reify 'the facts' as though they exist independently of interpretation, contextualisation and analysis, or as though they ought to function as unilateral determinants of social reality.

While the proposition of negotiated safety derived its authority from its demonstration through quantitative analysis, the second thing to notice is that the ability to interpret these data and produce the relevant analyses was very much predicated on relays between multiple forms of data. It simply would not have been possible to articulate negotiated safety without drawing upon other research techniques that enabled researchers to gain insight into the lived experiences, embodied meanings and practical logics of gay sex. In health policy circles, lip service is often paid to the desirability of qualitative research, where it seems to feature as a quaint pastime that might provide a bit of local colour and humanist sympathy. This is very different to how NCHSR researchers made use of qualitative research. Quantitative research-ers would actively solicit the findings of qualitative research and test the insights that emerged, almost doggedly, in their analyses of the distributive patterns and correlations within the quantitative data. Latour might describe this as a particular articulation – a way of arranging heterogenous sources of knowledge – in which the findings of one set of methods become engaged in the destiny and fate of many others. This is not a case of every approach hav-ing different but equally valid perspectives on the same object. Rather, the process of trialling, testing and articulating the findings of different method-ologies in relation with each other *produces new objects* through the installation of 'hybrid forums' (Callon, Lascoumes & Barthe 2009) in which various ver-sions of reality produce friction for, are made to animate and create questions for one another.

In the field of public health it is common to reify survey data and treat it as though it speaks for itself – 'the facts', pure and simple. But NCHSR researchers were always careful to insist that quantitative data must be interpreted much like qualitative data. Rather than providing inferential certainty, the patterns found in quantitative data were to be *interpreted* and theorised, drawing on the insights of social theory, and tested against other sources of knowledge. This conviction informed their commitment to more participatory forms of articulation. Since facts are always interpretations that cannot be read off the data transparently, it is important to try to be explicit about these interpretations and make them and their logics accessible to affected parties. Perhaps what impressed me most about the practices of the NCHSR was the extent to which practitioners of various persuasions – community, government, academia – were actively enrolled in methodological and interpretative debate about survey findings (even those with little quantitative training). NCHSR researchers actively fostered such engagements, translating their insights into a variety of epistemic formats. Nothing is predictable about scientific findings. Everything depends on the local interjections and practical interactions that shape the process of constructing them. These interactions shape what comes to matter in the process of scientific analysis. If facts are negotiable encounters, as my analysis suggests, this marks out a particularly active role for all those concerned. For facts are the scene where realities get made, meanings get fixed, and subjects are grasped as objects, their capacities circumscribed. 'Good science' exposes itself to specific trials of contestation, so that more realities are registered and the world becomes more interesting, provocative and differentiated for all those who are prepared to allow themselves to be affected by such encounters.

Thus while NCHSR researchers generally subscribed to the imperatives of evidence-based policy, their practices had the effect of querying these regimes of evidence from within. This became possible by giving 'due consideration to the particular object being studied, and . . . paying attention to the type of study design or analysis required to understand that object' (Kippax & Stephenson 2005, p. 361). The acknowledged complexity of sexual practice gave rise to articulations of research that engaged many actors in the making of the relevant facts. This made it possible to challenge prevailing moral and scientific orthodoxies on the basis of compelling evidence, which on this account can no longer mean the sort of evidence that is arrived at dutifully through the rote application of scientific procedures and established categories, but rather a social scientific approach that takes the risk of staging encounters with those who are most affected by its entry into the world. Such encounters become the occasion for mutually transformative relations in which the prehensions of science and those of the objects it engages are moved in unpredictable but consequential ways. Such encounters may be experienced as dreadful or delightful, worrisome or gay, indifferent or mobilising, depending on the manner in which they are entered into and what is made of them. As Despret puts it, '*We are allowed to speak interestingly by what we allow to speak interestingly'* (cited in Latour 1999, p. 144, emphasis in original). Conceived as events, research encounters become more generative and original.

Negotiated safety became something of a hallmark in Australian HIV education, enacting a distinct mode of attentiveness to the agency of sexual subjects in their dealings with the virus. Following its example, researchers later examined how gay men were incorporating new tests and treatments into their sexual repertoires (Rosengarten, Race & Kippax 2000; Kippax & Race 2003; Race 2003). Together, we were among the first to articulate a number of other risk-reduction strategies that made use of the perceived affordances of new antiretroviral therapies (Rosengarten, Race & Kippax 2000; Van de Ven et al. 2002, 2005; Race 2003). The point of these investigations was not simply to endorse these risk-reduction strategies in a blanket fashion, but to acknowledge these practices, suspend categorical judgement and initiate some sort of collective response to them. In this way, we hoped sexual players might become better equipped to make sense of the situations in which they might find themselves, and more sensible to the differences animating the sexual field at the time these studies were undertaken.

To note the finding of negotiated safety and recognise its prescience (only a decade later would US agencies begin to consider recognising similar practices) is to register a significant contribution to knowledge. But to frame it in this way gives little insight into the *doing* of social science, the sorts of encounters and relations through which such innovations became possible. It is hard to imagine the work of the NCHSR without recalling the diverse team of interlocutors it assembled within the course of its everyday practice: epidemiologists, community educators, people living with HIV, sex workers, drug-users, bureaucrats, doctors, etc. Each of these differently situated players became actively enlisted and engaged in making science through a variety of formal and informal arrangements. Thus, while the centre's directors always insisted on a clear distinction between science, community and government, to separate their contribution to knowledge from the experience of being involved in a broader social movement or 'partnership approach' misses something important about these scientific activities. There were moments of insight and occasional stoushes in meeting rooms and offices; unexpected convergences and laughter and difficult exchanges at committee meetings or with community advocates, doctors and bureaucrats at conferences; niggling intuitions and imaginative connections during hallway conversations; banter and discussion between researchers and community educators; rapid recruitment of people and resources around emerging issues; meticulous analysis of collected data and ongoing debate about research methods. Such dynamics could well be a feature of how science is generally done, though normally omitted from the pages of scientific journals. What distinguished this research culture was its preparedness to draw on such encounters and affirm the insights they generated to make social science strong enough to challenge certain orthodoxies.

The limits of control

I earlier named as *gay* a particular practical orientation to the world: one that takes delight in the unexpected; that finds a certain pleasure in contingency and movement; that attunes itself to the world's lively and eventful nature; that allows itself to be altered by its chance encounters and surprises. On the basis of this definition, I would argue there was something gay about the approach to HIV research developed by NCHSR researchers that has less to do with the sexuality of any member of this research team than the collective interest they took in the unexpected ways in which those they studied confounded established categories of analysis (definitions of risk and safe sex, for example).[5] This in turn led NCHSR researchers to problematise their analytic categories to remain responsive to what was happening in the field of sexual practice and devise new protocols of HIV prevention in conversation with the community sector and government. This represents an altogether different approach to the governance of risk within HIV prevention than that adopted within the US over the same period. For example, the US Centers for Disease Control and Prevention (CDC)'s Diffusion of Effective Behavioral Interventions, which structures the work of HIV service organisations in the USA, draws on the paradigm of evidence-based medicine to evaluate, standardise and coordinate behavioural interventions (Dworkin et al. 2008).[6] At the centrepiece of this programme is the use of the randomised controlled trial (RCT) to assess behavioural interventions. But this practice was criticised and contested by NCHSR researchers. In a series of important publications, NCHSR researchers rejected the appropriateness of RCTs for evaluating sexual health interventions (Kippax & Van de Ven 1998; Van de Ven & Aggleton 1999; Kippax 2003; Kippax & Stephenson 2005). Their basic argument is that control trials are unable to account for the complex processes through which social transformation occurs, which rarely take place over the short term, are never linear or unidirectional, and are always historically and culturally specific. Nor are the effects of a given intervention confined to isolated individuals.[7] As Kippax and Stephenson argue, 'complexity is *in* the object being studied and cannot be relegated to the role of external variables that can be studied independently, or that can be controlled for by invoking experimental design and method' (2005, p. 364).

Importantly, this rejection of controlled experiments does not imply giving up on rigorous evaluation. Rather, thick description of the social is advocated using a range of triangulated methods: cross-sectional and longitudinal surveys, qualitative studies, and the practical insights of affected communities. Here, data from a range of different sources is assembled and brought into articulation. While these articulations may not predict future change precisely as the RCT purports to do, 'they can help to understand the mechanisms through which change is occurring' (Kippax & Stephenson 2005, p. 366). On this view, it is a waste of time to obsess over predictability unless one expects society to remain the same, which it does not. Instead, it is necessary to solicit the interpretations of what is happening from those most affected by staging events that provide the conditions for what might be called *mutually transformative articulation*. The upshot of this work was to instantiate an alternative way of governing HIV that takes the critical step of dispensing with predictability in favour of responsiveness.

Latour regards scientific arrangements and practices as some of the key mechanisms through which we 'learn to be affected, meaning "effectuated", moved, put into motion by other entities, human or non-human' (2004a, p. 205), and we might usefully apply this insight to the governmentality of HIV. When viewed through this lens, the well-worn policy phrase 'communities affected by HIV' might start to give rise to a series of further interesting, important but seldom-asked questions, such as *how* are they/we affected, and what do given scientific practices and arrangements have to do with this? What hybrid forums might be assembled to better incorporate and produce scientific findings? To be sure, good HIV social science can stave off moral panic and temper sensationalistic responses, intervening in the overblown affects of moral hysteria, as I discuss in Chapter 4. But social science can also serve to attune us to important differences in sexual and prevention repertoires and practices, allowing us to 'become sensible to' more bodies, more affections, more realities; inviting us to become *more interested in* the differences that animate the sexual field as it is practised. While this facet of HIV social research poses certain challenges for education, the alternative is a rote insistence on behavioural norms that have an increasingly tenuous connection with people's actual practices and sense-making processes. Against this set of possibilities, *The Gay Science* aims to enact HIV prevention as a meaningful activity, meaning 'fluid, embedded in specific social formations' (Kippax & Stephenson 2005) and capable of sparking reflexive activity.

Changing infrastructures of gay life: a user's guide

The urban centres that became epicentres of gay life in the late twentieth century have undergone significant changes over the past two decades. The historical period this book engages is characterised by wide-ranging changes in the sociomaterial infrastructures of sex between men. A key change has been the introduction and widespread uptake of the Internet and other digital devices (such as smartphone apps) as prominent mechanisms for arranging sex between men. These devices have had concrete impacts on forms of sexual sociability, HIV prevention practices and relations among participants in gay sexual and social cultures: they represent a new infrastructure of the sexual encounter. They have also provided a platform for the invention and circulation of new sexual and risk identities, such as the barebacker, the 'chemsex' enthusiast, the Truvada whore and the [+u] online cruiser.[8] I call these socio-technical assemblages *digital infrastructures*.

As several of the new identities just noted also indicate, recent pharmaceutical developments have meant that the growing popularity of digital sex has been accompanied by significant changes in the corporeality and bioactivity of bodies. There have also been significant changes in practices of drug consumption (both medicinal and illicit) within gay sexual scenes. I describe these as transformations in *chemical infrastructures*. A third set of changes concerns the cultural geography of gay life and, in particular, the gradual but steady decline in the frequency with which gay men attend gay social and sexual venues that has occurred in many Western contexts (bars, clubs, dance parties, beats and urban streetscapes). As I go on to discuss, these changes can be attributed to a complex range of factors. I refer to them as changes in *communal infrastructures*.

The significance of these changing infrastructures of gay life for HIV prevention will become apparent in the chapters that together make up this book. Each set of developments has had wide-ranging impacts on how HIV prevention is *done*, prompting and necessitating innovations in HIV programming. Conceiving these developments in terms of changes to various overlapping, interpenetrating, converging and sometimes mutually interfering infrastructures is meant to signal the importance of devising more-than-human approaches for HIV analysis (see Whatmore 2006). These infrastructures change the terms through which people and things associate with each other, form bonds, dissociate, become sensitised to, ignore or avoid each other, providing the material support for different forms of sexual sociability at different moments. But like most infrastructures, they tend to serve some people better than others. Nor is their operation always reliable or exactly predictable, making the upsets they cause and our capacity to respond to them an active question.

A recurring theme throughout the book is the relation between sex and drug practices in their many forms: the sorts of transformations they have undergone; what each have made possible for the other; the differences they make to material situations and capacities; and how one might attend to their risks and pleasures constructively. Preciado (2013) has discussed how the rapid developments in global media and biotechnology that have animated advanced techno-capitalism since the mid-twentieth century have produced wide-ranging transformations in sex, gender, bodies, identities, sexuality and pleasure, referring to this period as 'the pharmacopornographic era'. This book investigates how to do 'counterpublic health' in such an era (Race 2009), and proposes some alternative ways of grasping what is happening and what might be done about it.

In terms of its structure, Chapters 2–6 of this book investigate how MSM have been made into responsible subjects of HIV prevention and harm reduction at different historical moments and through different assemblages. It explores some of the historical and sociotechnical infrastructures through which these processes have taken place (including the infrastructures of online cruising), their unexpected twists and turns and the resistance they have encountered. Chapters 7–9 move towards a much more explicit focus on the digital environments that have come to constitute much of the infrastructure for sexual encounters between men these days, exploring how these infrastructures are reconfiguring sex and drug practices and associated forms of sociability and community, and how they are being problematised. Digital mechanisms such as online cruising sites and smartphone apps have remediated the terms in which gay men encounter each other, search for sexual partners and associate with each other. I explore the implications of these developments for HIV prevention, harm reduction, counterpublic health and gay life, and propose some more affirmative ways of grasping and acting on these processes.

Finally, rather than imagining all these transformations to have taken place at arm's length from HIV science, in some mutually agreeable arrangement of externality, it should be clear by now that I understand scientific practices to be intimately and unpredictably entangled with the sexual and other practices they generally claim merely to describe and analyse. In this respect, scientific arrangements can be situated as the fourth infrastructure this book grapples with. My problematisation of different scientific practices in several chapters is undertaken with a view to realising some key principles of what I characterise as a gay science.

Notes

1 For the idea that drug use is merely an attempt to 'produce transformations', I am indebted to Stengers and Ralet (1997).
2 This conception will be elaborated in the chapters that follow (especially Chapter 5), but in the meantime see Latour (1999, p. 306) and Stengers (2000, p. 67).
3 If 'discovery' conceives a passive nature awaiting the application of human categories to make some sort of sense, 'event' anticipates constructivist attention to the agency of objects and their relations in processes of creativity and sociomaterial transformation. As Bruno Latour puts it, 'an event has consequences for the historicity of all the ingredients, including nonhumans, that are the circumstances of that experiment' (1999, p. 306).
4 Certainly, not all behavioural scientists working in Australia placed the same emphasis on this distinction, and a number of psychosocial scientists working outside the National Centre adopted behaviourist and biopsychological approaches.
5 It would be incorrect to assume NCHSR researchers were predominantly gay men. While a number of self-identified gay men did form part of this research team, just as crucial were the contributions made by heterosexual female and male and lesbian researchers to the research programme directed by Susan Kippax from 1990 until her retirement in 2008.
6 See Green (2016) for an excellent critical overview of this programme.
7 While NCHSR researchers held that drugs are more suitable for randomised evaluation, thus enacting a distinction between social and biomedical experiments, it could be argued that drugs have a complex agency, with effects extending well beyond the individual body to effectuate social, cultural and material transformations (Race 2009, pp. 51–4). In Chapter 6 I argue that this point calls for renewed practices of responsive attentiveness.
8 [+u] is an online identifier used by some HIV-positive individuals to indicate undetectable viral load (see Holas 2016).

References

Ahmed, S. 2010a. Killing joy: Feminism and the history of happiness. *Signs*, 35(3), pp. 571–594.

Ahmed, S. 2010b. *The Promise of Happiness*. Durham: Duke University Press.

Babich, B. 2006. Nietzsche's 'gay' science. In K. Ansell-Pearson (ed.) *A Companion to Nietzsche*. Chichester: Wiley-Blackwell, pp. 97–114.

Callon, M., Lascoumes, P. & Barthe, Y. 2009. *Acting in an Uncertain World*. Trans. G. Burchell. Cambridge: MIT Press.

Caserio, R., Edelman, L., Halberstam, J. et al. 2006. The antisocial thesis in queer theory. *PMLA*, 121(3), pp. 819–828.

Dworkin, S., Pinto, R., Hunter, J. et al. 2008. Keeping the spirit of community partnerships alive in the scale up of HIV/AIDS prevention: Critical reflections on the roll out of DEBI (diffusion of effective behavioral interventions). *American Journal of Community Psychology*, 42(1–2), pp. 51–59.

Ekstrand, M., Stall, R., Kegeles, S. et al. 1993. Safer sex among gay men: What is the ultimate goal? *AIDS*, 7(2), pp. 281–282.

Escoffier, J. 1998. The invention of safer sex: Vernacular knowledge, gay politics and HIV prevention. *Berkeley Journal of Sociology*, 43, pp. 1–30.

Foucault, M. 1984. *The History of Sexuality: An Introduction*. Trans. R. Hurley. London: Penguin Books.

Foucault, M. 1990. *The Use of Pleasure: Volume 2 of the History Of Sexuality*. Trans. R. Hurley. New York: Vintage Books.

Foucault, M. 1997a. Sex, power and the politics of identity. In P. Rabinow (ed.) *Ethics: Subjectivity and Truth*. London: Penguin, pp. 163–174.

Foucault, M. 1997b. Friendship as a way of life. In P. Rabinow (ed.) *Ethics: Subjectivity and Truth*. London: Penguin, pp. 135–140.

Foucault, M. 2011. The gay science. *Critical Inquiry*, 37(3), pp. 385–403.

Fraser, M. 2010. Facts, ethics and event. In C. Jensen & K. Rodje (eds.) *Deleuzian Intersections in Science, Technology and Anthropology*. Oxford: Berghahn Books, pp. 57–82.

Green, A. 2016. Keeping gay and bisexual men safe: The arena of HIV prevention science and praxis. *Social Studies of Science*, 46(2), pp. 210–235.

Gregg, M. 2006. *Cultural Studies' Affective Voices*. London: Palgrave MacMillan.

Halewood, M. 2011. *A.N. Whitehead and Social Theory: Tracing a Culture of Thought*. London: Anthem Press.

Halperin, D. 2011. Michel Foucault, Jean Le Bitoux, and the gay science lost and found: An introduction. *Critical Inquiry*, 37(3), pp. 371–380.

Hodges, M. 1980. *Flash Gordon*. Hollywood: Universal Pictures.

Holas, N. 2 January 2016. A gay's guide to undetectable. *Gay News Network* [online]. Retrieved from http://gaynewsnetwork.com.au/checkup/hiv/a-gay-s-guide-to-undetectable-17870.html [20 January 2017].

Kippax, S. 2003. Sexual health interventions are unsuitable for experimental evaluation. In J. Stephenson, J. Imrie & C. Bonell (eds.) *Effective Sexual Health Interventions: Issues in Experimental Evaluation*. Oxford: Oxford University Press, pp. 17–34.

Kippax, S., Crawford, J., Davis, M. et al. 1993. Sustaining safe sex: A longitudinal study of a sample of homosexual men. *AIDS*, 7(2), pp. 257–264.

Kippax, S. & Kinder, P. 2002. Reflexive practice: The relationship between social research and health promotion in HIV prevention. *Sex Education*, 2(2), pp. 91–104.

Kippax, S. & Race, K. 2003. Sustaining safe practice: Twenty years on. *Social Science & Medicine*, 57(1), pp. 1–12.

Kippax, S. & Stephenson, N. 2005. Meaningful evaluation of sex and relationship education. *Sex Education*, 5(4), pp. 359–373.

Kippax, S. & Van de Ven, P. 1998. An epidemic of orthodoxy? Design and methodology in the evaluation of the effectiveness of HIV health promotion. *Critical Public Health*, 8(4), pp. 371–386.

Latour, B. 1999. *Pandora's Hope*. London: Harvard University Press.

Latour, B. 2004a. How to talk about the body? The normative dimension of science studies. *Body & Society*, 10(2–3), pp. 205–229.

Mauss, M. 1973. Techniques of the body. *Economy and Society*, 2(1), pp. 70–88.

Michael, M. 2012. 'What are we busy doing?' Engaging the idiot. *Science, Technology & Human Values*, 37(5), pp. 528–554.

National Gallery of Art. 2016. *The Thinker (Le Penseur)* [online]. Retrieved from http://www.nga.gov/content/ngaweb/Collection/art-object-page.1005.html [17 January 2017].

Nietzsche, F. 2001. *The Gay Science*. Trans. J. Nauckhoff. Cambridge: Cambridge University Press (Orig. 1882).

Pippin, R. 2000. Gay science and corporeal knowledge. *Nietzsche Studien*, 29, pp. 136–152.

Preciado, P. 2013. *Testo-Junkie: Sex, Drugs, and Biopolitics in the Pharmacopornographic Era*. New York: The Feminist Press at CUNY.

Rabinow, P. 2005. Midst anthropology's problems. In A. Ong & S. Collier (eds.) *Global Assemblages: Technology, Politics, and Ethics as Anthropological Problems*. Oxford: Blackwell, pp. 40–54.

Race, K. 2003. Revaluation of risk among gay men. *AIDS Education & Prevention*, 15(4), pp. 369–381.

Race, K. 2008. The use of pleasure in harm reduction: Perspectives from *The History of Sexuality*. *International Journal of Drug Policy*, 19(5), pp. 417–423.

Race, K. 2009. *Pleasure Consuming Medicine*. Durham: Duke University Press.

Rosengarten, M., Race, K. & Kippax, S. 2000. *'Touch Wood, Everything Will Be Ok': Gay Men's Understandings of Clinical Markers in Sexual Practice*. Sydney: National Centre in HIV Social Research, UNSW.

Stengers, I. 2000. *The Invention of Modern Science*. Minneapolis: University of Minnesota Press.

Stengers, I. 2008. A constructivist reading of process and reality. *Theory, Culture & Society*, 25(4), pp. 91–110.

Stengers, I. & Ralet, O. 1997. Drugs: Ethical choice or moral consensus. In I. Stengers (ed.) *Power and Invention: Situating Science*. Minneapolis: University of Minnesota Press, pp. 215–232.

Van de Ven, P. & Aggleton, P. 1999. What constitutes evidence in HIV/AIDS education? *Health Education Research*, 14(4), pp. 461–471.

Van de Ven, P., Kippax, S., Crawford, J. et al. 2002. In a minority of gay men, sexual risk practice indicates strategic positioning for perceived risk reduction rather than unbridled sex. *AIDS Care*, 14(4), pp. 471–480.

Van de Ven, P., Mao, L., Fogarty, A. et al. 2005. Undetectable viral load is associated with sexual risk taking in HIV serodiscordant gay couples in Sydney. *AIDS*, 19(2), pp. 179–184.

Whatmore, S. 2006. Materialist returns: Practising cultural geography in and for a more-than-human world. *Cultural Geographies*, 13(4), pp. 600–609.

Whitehead, A. N. & Sherburne, D. 1981. *A Key to Whitehead's Process and Reality*. Chicago: University of Chicago Press.

Young, I. M. 1980. Throwing like a girl: A phenomenology of feminine body comportment motility and spatiality. *Human Studies*, 3(1), pp. 137–156.

2   Queer chemistry

Gay partying and collective innovations in care

Understanding the emergence of contemporary gay culture and political identity is impossible without considering the history of parties. A party is an event: a festive mode of social participation, a provisional and temporary coming together of diverse elements, people and things which creates new possibilities or makes something new emerge (that is, if you're lucky enough). Neither temporally permanent nor spatially fixed, parties nevertheless leave their imprint on cultural memory, urban geography and even political identity. While party practices are immensely variable and historically diverse, patterns can be traced which reveal much about the shifting relations between sexual minorities, social authorities and cultural economies. In *Pleasure Consuming Medicine*, I argued that greater attentiveness to pleasure and its varieties and social dynamics might enable us to devise new protocols and practices of care (Race 2009). Here, I want to extend that analysis with a more historically and geographically specific investigation of parties as they have featured in the formation and imagination of urban gay identity, with a particular focus on Sydney and some of the metropolitan histories its gay community habitually references such as those of New York.

This chapter sets the historical scene that constitutes the material and geographic backdrop to many of the analyses undertaken in this book. Its analysis stems from my interest in how modes of sexual sociability haven given rise to innovations in care practices historically. But I also want to situate partying as a significant communal infrastructure for gay life. Nightlife can be approached as a pedagogical space in which people learn to appreciate and take pleasure in difference through forms of interclass contact (Delany 1999) that transform subjectivities. Illicit drugs have been a significant component of the forms of sexual sociability this chapter discusses. This is not to say that all gay men do drugs, or that illicit drug use is a feature of homosexuality in general, but that drugs have been a significant component in the subcultural practices and spaces of pleasure upon which urban gay identity has been built. Of course gays, lesbians, queers and transgender people have made use of many different spaces to find each other in the heteronormative context. But bars, parties and nightclubs have played a special role as agents of gay socialisation (Southgate & Hopwood 1999; Green 2003).

The materialisation of gay political identity would not have been possible without drawing from the urban gay subcultures that constituted it as a recognisable source of collective identity.

While many studies have noted the association between gay social venues and drug use – usually as a problem for public health (Stall & Wiley 1988; Lewis & Ross 1995; Halkitis, Parsons & Stirratt 2001) – few have explored the part played by drug practices in the pleasures, identities and cultures that have emerged from them. A key claim of this chapter is that psychostimulant drugs have played a productive part in the materialisation of gay political identity in the twentieth century, serving as one of the chemical infrastructures of gay life. But how does one figure the significance of drug activity within social and cultural transformations? Grasping chemistry as a meaningful cultural force requires us to situate drugs as contingent players within particular sociocultural assemblages (Gomart & Hennion 1998; Malins 2004). Hence my focus on party practices. Situating drug use as one practice among the many that make up lives and cultures enables some acknowledgement of their activity in the formation and transformation of spaces of sexual expressivity without reifying drugs as fixed in terms of their significance or effects.

Pleasure, escape and gay sociability

The city is by now well recognised as a significant component in the emergence of modern gay identities and communities (D'Emilio 1983; Chauncey 1994; Bell & Binnie 2000; Eribon 2004). The journey to urban centres on the part of sexual outsiders can be understood in (at least) two ways: as an escape from oppressive heteronormative contexts, and as part of a search for sexual partners and sexual community (Delany 1999; Muñoz 2009). From the beginning of the twentieth century, cities such as New York, Berlin, Paris, London and Sydney have featured as 'elsewheres' in the homosexual imagination – safe havens where fellow sexual outsiders might be found. In the context of stigmatised identity, the mix of anonymity and critical mass found in cities has afforded many queer individuals a greater sense both of individual freedom and community. Where some scholars have considered the forms of stranger sociability and erotic attraction that characterise the city as 'precisely the obverse of community' (Young 1990, p. 239), it is possible to appreciate in this context how erotic pleasure has featured as the very *basis* of community. But this is assembled community – not the taken-for-granted community of transparent recognition that is thought to condition heterosexual self-formation. And the forms of pleasure that animate this community are themselves textured by the structures of the city. Thus for Henning Bech, 'the city is not merely a stage on which a pre-existing, preconstructed sexuality is displayed and acted out; it is also a space where sexuality is generated' (Bech 1997, p. 118).

A similar ambiguity around escape versus pleasure characterises explanations of drug use within gay and lesbian populations. Just as movement to the city could be understood in terms of escape from an oppressive normative order, drugs have been understood as a means of escaping cognitive awareness of oppressive norms around sexual identity and sexual practice (McKirnan, Ostrow & Hope 1996). In *The Boys in the Band* (Crowley 1969), the theatrical depiction of a birthday party among gay friends in a New York loft, one of the characters coins the 'Christ-was-I-drunk-last-night syndrome' to discuss the ways in which alcohol can be used to mediate the stigma and shame around homosexuality:

> You know, when you made it with some guy in school, and the next day when you had to face each other there was always a lot of shit-kicking crap about, "Man, was I drunk last night! Christ, I don't remember a thing!"
>
> (Crowley 1969, p. 41)

Though initially discussed among the gay friends at the party as a ploy that closeted youth use to justify homosexual activities 'after the event', in the discussion that ensues it becomes evident that it may take the shape of a more deliberate and widespread strategy. So when Michael expands:

> You see, in the Christ-was-I-drunk-last-night syndrome, you really *are* drunk. That part of it is true. It's just that you also *do remember everything*. [General laughter]. Oh God, I used to have to get loaded to go in a gay bar!
>
> (1969, p. 42)

Another guest responds, '[a] lot of guys have to get loaded to have sex' (p. 43), depicting intoxication less as a loss of control than a deliberate – if less than ideal – sexual strategy.

This use of alcohol to mediate intensities of guilt, stigma and shame in relation to homosexual practice and identity might be read as a product of the times (and indeed one reviewer of the film based on the play complained of the characters' 'self-lacerating vision of themselves [which] belongs to another time' (Guthmann 1999)). This interpretation finds support in much of the sociological literature, which attributes homosexual substance use to depression, alienation and the stigmatised status of homosexuality (Stall & Wiley 1988; Lewis & Ross 1995; Halkitis et al. 2001). But the involvement of alcohol in the course of the drama suggests that intoxication also played a part in the genres of banter, rivalry, play, confrontation, disclosure and affective exchange which characterised the elaboration of (some) gay friendship networks in this context. A focus on the pleasures afforded by intoxicants, however temporary and ambiguous these may appear, may give some insight into the experiential shape and texture of particular social worlds and the conditions in which participants attempt certain transformations or escapes.

The slightly maudlin depiction of gay intoxication offered by *The Boys in the Band* can be set alongside novels such as Ford and Tyler's (1933)

The Young and Evil or Andrew Holleran's (1978) *The Dancer from the Dance*, which lyrically depict the gay social and party scenes of New York in the 1930s and 1970s respectively. Here, intoxicants appear to be indispensably involved in the expressivity of an entire subculture and set of practices: the drug-saturated disco culture of Holleran's (1978) novel, for example, with its exuberant and distinctive practices of dance, glamour, friendship, music and sex. Drugs are everywhere in this text – poppers, angel dust, amphetamines, cocaine, Quaaludes, valium, alcohol – but they are generally subordinated to the pleasures of context:

> Some of the dancers are on drugs and enter the discotheque with the radiant faces of the Magi coming to the Christ Child; others, who are not, enter with a bored expression, as if this is the last thing they want to do tonight. In half an hour they are indistinguishable, sweat-stained, ecstatic, lost. For the fact was drugs were not necessary to most of us, because the music, youth, sweaty bodies were enough. . . . We lived for music, we lived for Beauty and we were poor.
>
> (Holleran 1978, p. 115)

While the disco culture depicted in *Dancer from the Dance* is unimaginable without drugs, drugs are dispersed as an ancillary component to the primary activities of dancing and sexual sociability. Meanwhile, dancing itself features as a means of elaborating social bonds which suspend the couple form, perhaps indefinitely:

> Now of all the bonds between homosexual friends, none was greater than that between friends who danced together. The friend you danced with, when you had no lover, was the most important person in your life; and for people who went without lovers for years, that was all they had. It was a continuing bond.
>
> (Holleran 1978, pp. 111–12)

No longer simply a mechanism to assuage guilt or enable sexual coupling, intoxication emerges as one aspect of a culture of playful participation and socio-sexual interaction that has a particularity of its own.

The depiction of drugs in *Dancer from the Dance* indicates the importance of considering the social organisation of urban gay life when accounting for homosexual drug use. It is inadequate to rely on explanations of social stigma alone. Yet it would be too simplistic to separate the motivation of escape from a more positive consideration of the contexts of pleasure altogether. Rather, what is needed is an appreciation of how the different sides of this polarity fold into one another at different moments in different lives, and how agencies of pleasure respond specifically to broader contexts of judgement and everyday, normative pressure. Indeed, in both these texts the use of intoxicating substances has an acknowledged complexity, featuring as an escape from overbearing normative standards, an opportunity for self-expression and self-justification, and a means of producing new contexts of sexual sociability and interaction that might otherwise be difficult to achieve.

With these considerations in mind, what follows is a discussion of some of the forms of public sociability that have been important in the formation of urban gay culture. Drugs and alcohol have been a significant part of these practices, sometimes incidentally (simply because they have gone with the territory) and sometimes in terms of their perceived capacity to conjure new materialities – the contexts of action and interaction I mentioned above. The practices of sexual sociability in which drugs and alcohol are bound up have attracted intense surveillance and intervention on the part of social authorities. These scenes of illicit sexuality and consumption have constituted key targets of disciplinary attempts to privatise and normalise sexuality. But they have also been incorporated into regimes of economic value, in official efforts to promote tourism and consumption in the 'post-liberation' context, for example. These contradictory investments in the scene of gay partying give drugs an ambiguous but volatile status within the regimes of consumer society, as I will later illustrate with reference to contemporary disputes around drug policing in Sydney.

Disorderly premises

> Respectable gays like to think that they owe nothing to the sexual subculture they think of as sleazy. But their success, their way of living, their political rights and their very identities would not have been possible but for the existence of the public sexual culture they now despise.
>
> (Berlant & Warner 1998, p. 563)

These comments from Berlant and Warner resonate with the sense in which formal political discourses tend to disavow or forget the (often messy, always complex) contribution of social and cultural events and dynamics to wide-scale transformations in the conditions of everyday life – transformations of great political and material significance. Though sometimes depicted as a phenomenon of post-Stonewall consumer culture, the significance of parties and partying for gay sexual sociability precedes and exceeds the relatively short history of gay liberation. Historically excluded from some of the key institutions of private life, such as marriage and the family, homo-erotically inclined men have long made use of public and semi-public venues – such as bars, coffee shops, parties, parks, public restrooms, bookstores and bathhouses – to meet other men and pursue social and sexual ties. George Chauncey depicts a thriving urban gay culture spread out across a host of commercial establishments, social events, dance events and public spaces in New York, even before the 1920s (Chauncey 1994). More locally, the attraction of many single men to the city led to the concentration of identifiably homosexual clientele in some city pubs and bars as early as the 1920s and 1930s in Sydney, while the influx of servicemen during World War II boosted the clientele of these venues and led to the emergence of Kings Cross as a key nightlife district with a growing homosexual presence (Wotherspoon 1991).

Not surprisingly, the legal prohibition of homosexuality meant that public gathering spots and venues frequented by gay men were subject to frequent police raids. In his history of the gay subculture in Sydney, Gary Wotherspoon (1991) provides an account from a patron of Black Ada's, a popular underground nightclub based in an old dance studio in the city in the 1930s:

> The place was packed to the hilt, dim lights, a bottle of 'plonk', lots of 'knowall' girls as a front and in the half light everyone looked beautiful. The dancing was real, body to body, pre-war stuff and you haven't lived unless you've really danced – asking some beaut guy for a dance, clasping him in your arms and cheek to cheek – sex on the dancefloor! About 1am the Vice Squad used to make its routine call and when Black Ada opened the door and saw them she would press a bell and we'd all scatter for our seats leaving only the blokes dancing with the girls. So by the time the Vice Boys got to the top of the stairs it looked like a Sunday School hop and Ada used to call out in time to the music, 'one, two, turn – one, two. Will the couple on the right keep in step!' We all pissed ourselves at the tables trying to look as if we were studying the waltz.
>
> (cited in Wotherspoon 1991, p. 61)

Though it became increasingly popular over the course of World War II, the Vice Squad soon closed Black Ada's, considering it too 'corrupting' an influence to leave open.

Parties and balls were one of the more conspicuous forms of socialising among Sydney's homo-erotically inclined men and their friends (Wotherspoon 1991). Parties relied on extended friendship networks and were often hastily arranged before city pubs closed at 6pm. Balls were more elaborate affairs, some even being held annually in public halls. Some of the bigger parties such as the Drag and Drain parties of the 1930s and 40s and Artist and Models Balls of the 1950s and 60s catered to a wider bohemian set, with drag and cross-dressing regularly featuring. These were exuberant affairs by all accounts: Wotherspoon writes of drag queens arriving in removal vans, since their gowns and wigs were so elaborate that there was no other way to get there (1991, p. 135). When police harassment and surveillance of homosexual activity reached a peak in the context of the Cold War, these private and semi-public parties took on a new significance in sustaining Sydney's homosexual subcultures. Organisers now had to go to extreme lengths to avoid police detection, including selling tickets only very close to the event, refusing to sell tickets to unknown guests, meeting at suburban train stations and organising travel to the dancehall from there. While constant police harassment eventually forced many of them to be abandoned, these larger-scale events were in many ways the precursors of Sydney's giant dance parties of the

1980s, which were largely responsible for popularising dance music and the drug ecstasy in Australia.

In his history of New York's gay community, Chauncey shows how the alcoholic beverage control laws developed after Prohibition in the 1930s expanded the state's ability to regulate public sociability with a profound impact on urban gay sociality (Chauncey 1994). Where Prohibition had transformed the boundaries of acceptable public sociability by allowing an unanticipated intermingling of the classes and sexes in the underground demimonde of the speakeasy (precisely the opposite of what was intended), the establishment of the State Liquor Authority as the exclusive authority for licensing the sale of alcohol in the post-Prohibition context led to a sanitisation of the nighttime environment which effectively suppressed public expressions of homosexual sociability. In particular, the mechanism of the licence made proprietors responsible (under threat of revocation of licence) for ensuring that premises did not become 'disorderly'. This gave authorities a new way to reinforce the boundaries of respectable public sociability by regulating the public spaces where people met to drink. While the legislature did not specifically prohibit bars from serving homosexuals, the New York State Liquor Authority made it clear in practice and numerous legal instances that the mere presence of gay men, lesbians, prostitutes, gamblers or other 'deviant' figures was enough to condemn an establishment as 'disorderly' and lead to a revocation of license. 'In the two and a half decades that followed, it closed literally hundreds of bars that welcomed, tolerated, or even failed to notice the patronage of gay men or lesbians' (Chauncey 1994, p. 339).

While there is less evidence of liquor licensing provisions being used in this way in Sydney, the constant police harassment of public and semi-public parties makes it possible to see how forms of public sociability involving the consumption of intoxicating substances have constituted a key target of disciplinary attempts to privatise and normalise sexuality more generally. The convergence of various regulatory operations around illicit sexuality, intoxication and public sociability reveals this site to be a nexus of some significance for understanding confrontations between regulatory power, social experimentation and queer resistance. But these prohibitive arrangements also suited certain entrepreneurial interests. The demand for gay social spaces in the context of illegality turned gay bars into very attractive propositions for organised crime. In Sydney, the illegal status of homosexuality enabled the development of close links between organised crime, corrupt police and the owners of gay commercial establishments, some of whom allegedly paid huge sums of money to operate (Faro 2000; Hurley 2001). In her 'true crime' account of relations between organised crime and gay commercial establishments in Sydney in the early 1980s, Harvey describes how Patch's – one of the first of the popular disco-style nightclubs designed to cater to a gay clientele on Oxford Street – allegedly contained a large wooden tea chest stuffed with cash used to pay off police (Harvey 2000, p. 124). The criminalisation of homosexuality created conditions fit for exploitation by a range of corrupt organisations.

A similar concentration of police surveillance, illicit gender and sexual expression, organised crime and underground consumption animated the events that precipitated the Stonewall Riots in 1969 in New York (commonly referred to as the birth of the modern LGBTIQ rights movement). Like many venues frequented by gender and sexual minorities at this time, the Stonewall Inn did not have a liquor licence but was owned and controlled by a mafia family, who were in the habit of paying off police to prevent raids (Duberman 1993). Police harassment and entrapment of these populations for solicitation was so intense over this period that bars had become one of the few places where gays, lesbians and transgender people could openly congregate in New York without being arrested. When police raided the Stonewall Inn one busy summer night, many patrons refused to produce their identification. Police responded with mass arrests. The crowd that gathered in Greenwich Village that night to witness these arrests soon broke out into a series of violent confrontations with police. The ensuing events are generally regarded as a catalyst for the more outspoken forms of gay activism that took shape in this period, which have been discussed extensively elsewhere (Adam 1987; Duberman 1993; Carter 2004). Among the sporadic protests undertaken by insurgents over the next few days was the distribution of a leaflet which read 'Get the Mafia and the Cops out of Gay Bars' – an indication of widespread frustration with prevailing regimes of underground consumption and surveillance (Duberman 1993, p. 205).

A magical and volatile formula

The emergence of a lucrative market for heterosexual prostitution in Sydney during the Vietnam War prompted a change in the spatial configuration of gay subcultural venues in that city (Faro 2000). In Kings Cross, where a nascent camp culture had gradually emerged, 'even the streets themselves, with their pimps, working women, and drunken, often abusive clients, were increasingly hostile to camp men' (Faro 2000, p. 223), and many businesses catering to a gay clientele turned their attention to nearby Oxford Street which became the site of a new, US-influenced, much more visible enactment of gay identity over the 1970s, complete with nightclubs, bars, US-themed cafes and sex venues. For gay men, a much more studied, masculinised, 'clone' look replaced the effeminacy which for so long had defined homosexual male subculture, while the popularity of groups such as the Village People was matched by the uptake of many of the accoutrements of disco, including amyl-nitrate poppers: 'the drug that defined an era, fuelling both the ecstatic twirl of the dancers at nightclubs and . . . sexual hedonism' (Faro 2000, p. 245).

Perhaps the event that most firmly consolidated Oxford Street as a place of political significance for gay culture was Mardi Gras, which began in 1978 as a procession commemorating the Stonewall Riots, but culminated in a violent clash with police leading to the arrest of fifty-three people. Mardi Gras grew into an annual street parade and massive party and one of Australia's most popular and distinctive public events. The history of Mardi Gras is complex and has been discussed extensively elsewhere (Marsh & Galbraith 1995; Carbery 1995; Haire 2001). Here I merely identify a number of features that may help contextualise the significance of party events in the materialisation of public gay identity in Australia.

The first of these is the way Mardi Gras successfully fused political activism with the forms of cultural recreation and subcultural pleasure which animated the emerging commercial gay scene. In the 1970s there was a perceived disjuncture between recreational participants in the bar and club scene and the more politically minded activists intent on social and legal reform, with some degree of mutual suspicion between these groups (Faro 2000). The first parade was designed as a form of 'political outreach', and the mix of fancy dress, dancing, marching and chanting distinguished it from more conventional genres of protest march. Chants such as 'out of the bars and onto the streets!' successfully attracted participants from among the Saturday night patrons on Oxford Street, boosting the scale of the protest event significantly. This formula was retained and expanded upon in later years with the addition of huge, irreverent, satirical floats designed by Sydney's queer artistic talent. The event was rescheduled to a night in summer to capitalise on the warmer, more festive atmosphere. As a later president of the organisation, Richard Cobden, emphasised over a decade later,

> in 1978 our community in Sydney happened across a magical and volatile formula – a political protest blended with in-your-face extravagance and creativity. The magic and volatility worked. We created a lesbian and gay protest quite unlike anything else in the world – a celebration.
>
> (Faro 2000, p. 236)

Whatever sentimentality might be evident in this analysis, it is clear that Mardi Gras provided a powerful source of collective identification for differently motivated gay, lesbian and transgender individuals. By bringing an innovative form of public and political expression to the city's streets that emphasised play and parodic performance, the history of the event belies leftist distinctions between political activism and consumer pleasure (Marsh & Galbraith 1995; Hurley 2001; Race 2009).

Second, Mardi Gras contributed to a culture of public partying that was participatory, spectacular and widely accessed. The dance parties associated with the event drew on many of the conventions of the drag balls of previous eras while taking them to a new degree of intensity and scale (Wotherspoon 1991; Faro 2000). Dance parties are often overlooked in political histories of Mardi Gras beyond their function as key fundraisers for the organisation. But these events became key sources of collective identification and popular involvement, uniquely implicated in elaborations of queer belonging. The Mardi Gras dance party was held in the enormous pavilions of the Royal Agricultural Showgrounds directly after the parade and soon came to attract crowds of over 15,000 people. While drug use was more obviously associated with the dance party than the parade, the event as a whole can be characterised in terms of a culture of public partying in which drug use featured as a widely acknowledged – if variably accessed –component. With multiple relays and intersections between the parade, the dance parties, and the commercial and street-based recovery parties that followed over the next few days, the Mardi Gras party was characterised by wider and more diverse forms of participation than perhaps is typical of the US 'circuit party'. Actively referencing as well as interweaving with the many other gay-friendly public parties that emerged in Sydney at this time (such as the RAT parties and Sleaze Ball),[1] Mardi Gras parties featured creative design concepts, individual themes, dance music, party drugs such as ecstasy, amphetamine and LSD, extravagant live performances, guest celebrities and audio-visual effects, and attracted thousands of gays, lesbians, drag queens and transgender participants as well many heterosexual bohemians (Faro 2000). With recorded electronic dance music spun by DJs, flamboyant display, the stimulation afforded by party drugs and gender experimentation, these parties contrasted sharply with the hetero-masculine pub rock scene of the 1980s mainstream and its drinking culture. Party drugs were a staple component of these events and were valued for their ability to construct new contexts of intimacy, eroticism, affection, play, expressivity, sensation and perception. The Mardi Gras parties and RAT parties started a craze for giant dance parties in Sydney that did much to transform the city's nightlife and general character by popularising gay-friendly dance music and associated practices.

The third aspect of Mardi Gras that deserves comment in this context is its unexpected impact on concepts and practices of public health. Mardi Gras made it possible to imagine new styles of public health that thematised community education and pleasure (Ballard 1992; Marsh & Galbraith 1995; Sendziuk 2003; Race 2009). At the beginning of the AIDS crisis in 1983–4 there were calls to ban the parade, with one of the government's principal advisors on AIDS describing the post-parade party as a 'Bacchanalian orgy' (Haire 2001, p. 101). What was at issue at this juncture was the strategy for responding to AIDS – a punitive legal and medical regime or community education, partnership and participation. A legal framework for the protection of civil rights had been enacted over the early 1980s, including anti-discrimination measures and the decriminalisation of homosexuality. The sense of a coherent, organised, identifiable community that Mardi Gras appeared to embody made it possible to imagine a 'community response to AIDS' – a phrase that soon worked its way into policy discourse and became a basis for further mobilisation. The transformation in consciousness was so effective that the same medical advisor reversed his position in 1985 to suggest that 'Mardi Gras would provide a perfect forum for large-scale education about AIDS' (Marsh & Galbraith 1995, p. 308).

Elsewhere I have written about the significance of the construct of 'community' for gay responses to HIV. The sense of community that was enacted at dance parties 'helped sustain a collective sense of predicament, power, care and commitment – a shared ethos enabling wide-ranging cooperation and transformative activity' (Race 2009, p. 22). This transformative activity included the invention and promotion of a safe-sex ethic and the creation and sustenance of friendship networks outside the family form which became so important in the context of the social exclusion, death and dying associated with AIDS. What is less frequently acknowledged is the participation of drugs such as ecstasy in the materialisation of this community response (Lewis & Ross 1995; Bardella 2002). The feelings of peace, empathy, openness and caring stimulated by ecstasy contributed to relational intensities, embodied dispositions and wider structures of feeling which for many gave further force, coherence and meaning to a whole range of caring and bonding activities. Indeed, recent clinical proposals to test drugs such as ecstasy and ketamine for their efficacy in treating post-traumatic stress disorder and depression may simply represent a more formalised version of some of the forms of collective experimentation that were taking place on gay dance floors over the 1980s and 90s in response, at least in part, to HIV/AIDS.

Of course, the organisation of dance parties raised challenges of its own, and it was in this context that further innovations in care practice developed. The participation of people with AIDS in the Mardi Gras dance parties in the early years of the crisis required the services of a medical tent, and organisers pulled together front-line volunteer teams of nurses, doctors, paramedics and first aiders to service these large-scale events (Masters 2007). The needs of HIV-positive patrons ranged from emotional support to feelings of illness, fatigue and other mishaps requiring rest and medical care. But the team was soon called upon to service a much more diverse range of presentations and needs, ranging from physical injuries to costume mishaps and, more topically, drug-related emergencies and accidents. The latter category of situations demanded a particular approach to care that was non-judgemental, responsive to circumstances and avoided moralism. Certain strategies were adopted, such as the exclusion of certain authorities from the medical tent (security officers, licensees or police) to maintain confidentiality and ensure effective communication and the safe treatment of patrons. With only a tiny percentage of patrons presenting for care requiring emergency transfer to local hospitals, the Mardi Gras medical tent pioneered a pragmatic and effective first-line health service that served as a model for drug harm reduction at dance events.

Later in its history, in response to the growing popularity of drugs such as Gamma-Hydroxybutyrate (GHB) at dance events, further innovations in care practice were devised by community agencies. When taken according to certain protocols, this drug is relatively innocuous, but when taken in too big a dose, or too frequently, or mixed with depressants such as alcohol, it can lead users to lose consciousness, which in some circumstances can result in serious consequences such as coma and/or death. In response to the increasing frequency of serious incidents at gay dance events, ACON NSW introduced the ACON Rovers, a team of community volunteers who rove around dance parties on the lookout for patrons in trouble. Since overdosing on GHB causes users to lose consciousness, such incidents often come to the attention of medical personnel too late. Described by its inventors as 'the eyes and ears of the medical tent', this initiative has achieved wide-ranging community support and proved remarkably effective in terms of preventing many of the casualties associated with use of GHB at LGBTIQ dance events (Gonçalves et al. 2016). It can be regarded as a further innovation in care practice emerging from within the communal infrastructure of party environments that openly fosters attention to the social pragmatics of drug use in this setting, its risks and its pleasures.

The final aspect of Mardi Gras that is relevant to this discussion is its contribution to Sydney's international reputation, such that in 2000 it could be described in a mainstream academic publication as a 'principal signifier of Sydney' where 'images of Sydney as exuberant (homo)sexuality become mainstream, as gay men and lesbians, alongside heterosexual couples, families, tourists and households, turn out to celebrate the city in its public spaces' (Gibson & Connell 2000, p. 308). This transformation in the public image of Sydney's sexual subcultures from a stigmatised and despised minority to a position of symbolic centrality in the city's international imaginary was nothing short of extraordinary. Indeed, local spectators watching the closing ceremony of Sydney Olympic Games in 2000 – with its giant floats, drag queens, pink-suited dancing boys and well-known gay icon pop singer Kylie Minogue – could not help being struck by the event's constant references and cultural indebtedness to the spectacular conventions of Sydney's urban queer subcultures (Markwell 2002).

There is some discussion in the critical literature of how state and municipal authorities appropriate counterpublic spaces to gear their urban landscapes to a consumer environment and reposition the city as a tourist magnet in the global economy (Quilley 1997; Hurley 2001; Haire 2001; Hobbs et al. 2003; Waitt & Markwell 2003; Bell & Binnie 2004). This literature is useful for understanding subsequent transformations in Sydney's urban spaces, as I will discuss in further detail. It is noteworthy, however, that the growth of Mardi Gras over this period occurred despite (rather than because of) the entrepreneurial activities of official tourism bodies. Notwithstanding the range of official efforts to refashion Australian cities as key players in the global economy through the promotion of hallmark events (mainly sports), Mardi Gras was tolerated at best and largely ignored by state authorities for almost two decades. Indeed, as late as 1990 the Minister for Tourism ordered the NSW Tourism Commission to remove material relating to Mardi Gras from its premises and databases on 'moral grounds' (Marsh & Galbraith 1995, p. 313). It was only in its third decade, after the commissioning of several economic impact statements by the organisation itself, that Mardi Gras came to be explicitly embraced and promoted on the basis of its impact on the regional economy (assessed to be greater than any other national hallmark event) (Haire 2001). Nevertheless, with its tendency to draw crowds of up to 750,000 people to the city streets to watch the parade, the event had successfully positioned itself as a lucrative commodity and tourist draw-card by the late 1990s, attracting significant commercial sponsorship and being broadcast on live television across the country and internationally and advertised in tourist promotions, with its cultural artefacts publicly exhibited in galleries, books and museums.

Perhaps one of the most remarkable cultural transformations associated with Mardi Gras is the changing relation between sexual minorities and the police – a relation which could be taken as a barometer of citizenship status. While traditionally relations between police and sexual minorities in Sydney had been extremely hostile, the organisers of the 1984 Mardi Gras became involved in efforts to establish direct liaison between police and emerging gay and lesbian organisations, as recommended in state anti-discrimination reports a few years earlier (Marsh & Galbraith 1995). Mardi Gras provided a key opportunity for brokering relationships between gay and lesbian organisers and the police: indeed cooperation and interaction with police was crucial in maintaining such a large-scale public event. Over the next few years participants reported a general improvement in relations with police and an increased acknowledgement within police circles of their role in supporting the event, despite some initial tensions. When the Sisters of Perpetual Indulgence, a satirical order of gay male nuns, decided to exorcise the Darlinghurst police station of 'the demon of homophobia' on its closure in 1987, the contingent of NSW police who gathered to watch the event did little but stand 'bemusedly looking on' (Faro 2000, p. 237). In 1990, the police gave Mardi Gras a community award for 'ongoing cooperation and crowd and safety control measures' (Marsh & Galbraith 1995, p. 317). In 1991 they started advertising in the Mardi Gras Guide. By 1998 they were marching in the parade. This was an extraordinary transformation in police–community relations. Over the 1990s, anti-violence initiatives tackling homophobia built on these relations, successfully interpellating police with LGBTIQ concerns and constituting LGBTIQ populations as legitimate recipients of state care rather than targets of state intervention and violence (Tomsen 2001). And while police were aware of the drug use associated with gay party culture over the 1990s (Southgate & Hopwood 1999), drug consumption did not constitute an explicit priority of public operations in the context of harm minimisation discourses that were prevalent over this period.

Step back in time

Shortly after Mardi Gras 2009, an opinion piece appeared in one of Sydney's gay and lesbian newspapers entitled 'Step Back in Time' (Sant 2009) in which lesbian barrister Kathy Sant argued that NSW police should be banned from marching in the Mardi Gras parade until hostile and oppressive police actions at gay and lesbian events ceased. In particular, Sant criticised the large police presence at the Mardi Gras party and the use of sniffer dogs to instigate searches of partygoers inside and outside the party. 'Lots of things are better in 2009 but for some reason the NSW police force has chosen to take a step back in time', Sant wrote. She went on to compare recent police operations to the violent confrontations of the first Mardi Gras:

> Just like in 1978, there was police hostility, harassment and unjustified violence (in the form of invasive searches) against innocent people. . . . There was roughly the same number of arrests as at the first Mardi Gras. Once again people were frightened about losing their jobs or damage to their reputations.
>
> (Sant 2009)

Sant's article elicited a wave of support in the letters pages, with many writers agreeing with her comments and criticising the police. This prompted a written response from Assistant Commissioner of Police Catherine Burn, who defended police actions on the night and constructed drug searches as a reasonable response to 'anti-social behavior' (Burn 2009). Pointing to the use of sniffer dogs at a number of recent music festivals and non-gay-specific dance parties, Burn rejected the idea that police operations were homophobically motivated or unfairly singled out gay and lesbian spaces. 'Drug possession is not just an offence, but drug use is dangerous and harmful to one's health and wellbeing', Burns wrote. 'There should be a focus on educating the community rather than condemnation of police for doing their job'.

The community outcry revealed much about the significance of party practices in the constitution and recreation of gay and lesbian identity in Sydney. While the police had conducted similar operations at non-gay raves and music festivals, rarely had they received such sustained and extensively voiced public criticism of them on the part of event participants. Notable here was the tacit community acknowledgement of the significance of drug practices in the viability of gay dance culture. While Mardi Gras itself disowned the drug use of participants, a former president of the organisation speculated in the gay press that 'Mardi Gras has faced serious crises during its 30 years, but this one [police use of sniffer dogs] has the potential to take down the organization once and for all' (McLachlan 2009). This exchange between police and their critics reveals how powerfully the drug raid reverberates with historical narratives and cultural memories of state intervention into queer social practices. By invoking the legacy of disciplinary attempts to suppress gay public sociability under the guise of regulating intoxicant consumption, critics constructed a powerful basis for resisting this instance of social government. But is this just another instance of homophobic state action, continuous with the past? Does identity politics provide a sufficient means of resisting and contesting these policing practices?

The threat posed to gay space by current practices of drug policing represents a new chapter in the government of liminal consumption. To understand these dynamics, we must consider the effects of the economic investment in gay spaces that has taken place in the contemporary consumer context – in particular, the emergence of the nighttime economy as a problematic object of government (Hobbs et al. 2003). Where previous interventions into the scene of gay partying targeted deviant expressions of sexuality and gender through direct police intervention and the mechanism of the licence, in this instance it would appear that queer social spaces have been caught up in the broader government of 'anti-social behaviour' and nighttime violence in a way that nonetheless threatens the existence of gay-friendly urban culture. Given the historical use of dance drugs to elaborate its particular modes of urban belonging, it is not surprising that gay community has become the locus of some of the most vocal objections to this policing strategy. But behind this drama is not simply homophobic policy but an inadequate analysis of the contingency of drug effects (Race 2014).

The 'antisocial behaviour' of police discourse

The extraordinary popularity of Mardi Gras by the end of the 1990s brought a greater volume of mainstream consumers to the recreational precincts of Oxford Street on weekend nights. Within the cultural narratives and marketing discourse associated with nighttime consumption, gay space offers various degrees of liminal experience: intrigue, excitement, transgression, novelty and adventure – a zone where day-time identities and norms can be momentarily suspended (Waitt & Markwell 2006; Race 2016). For sexual minorities, the marketing of this space to non-gay consumers and the increasing presence of heterosexuals within them can represent a loss of control over crucial zones of communal elaboration and produce a sense of disenfranchisement (Quilley 1997; Waitt & Markwell 2006). Indeed, the desexualisation of gay space within discourses of cultural economy and the loss of associated symbolic meanings is perfectly illustrated in the city branding discourse cited above, which depicts how 'images of Sydney as exuberant (homo)sexuality become mainstream, as gay men and lesbians, alongside heterosexual couples, families, tourists and households, turn out to celebrate the city in its public spaces' (Gibson & Connell 2000, p. 308).

The attraction of increased numbers of recreational consumers into the Oxford Street area on weekend nights brought with it many of the problems associated with the expansion of nighttime leisure in urban centres around the world more generally: violence and disorder, accident and injury, congestion, public drunkenness and so-called 'anti-social behaviour' (Hobbs et al. 2003). Further tensions surfaced after a spate of attacks on gay men in this late-night precinct were met with police inaction. While many within the gay community interpreted these attacks as homophobic, a broader discourse on public drunkenness, drug and alcohol-related violence and antisocial behaviour had developed in association with the expansion of nighttime leisure over the previous decade, and police interpreted the problems on Oxford Street largely through this lens.[2] Investigation of the homophobic dynamics of this violence became subsumed to the more predominant discourse of 'drug and alcohol-related violence'. Perhaps the best illustration of the paradoxical impact of this discourse came in 2007 when the Lord Mayor and the Minister for Police answered the call of a local drag identity to walk down Oxford Street on Saturday night to 'witness first-hand the nightly antisocial behaviour'. Police responded a couple of weekends later with Operation Gilligan's, a high-profile operation in which police took drug dogs through a number of venues on Oxford Street (gay and straight), leading to the arrest of several people for possessing drugs and the closure of the Manacle, one of the few remaining queer-friendly venues on the strip, for breaching its licensing conditions. Paradoxically, the equation of antisocial behaviour with illicit intoxication produced further assaults on gay-friendly social venues in this precinct.

Police attempted to justify the use of drug dogs in terms of confronting drug and alcohol-related violence and the illegality of drugs in general. But the conflation of drugs and alcohol in this discourse fails to think through the assemblages within which specific substances participate and their variable effects – the narratives, relations, affects, meanings, spaces and gendered performances with which they are entangled. The gay dance culture can be substantially and practically differentiated from the hetero-masculine drinking culture with which much nighttime violence is associated (Lewis & Ross 1995). Gay events are rarely places of in-group violence: in what could be described as a scene of liminal consumption *par excellence*, the Mardi Gras party attracts 20,000 people to public pavilions in inner Sydney yet few incidents of violence within party grounds are ever recorded. The coherence of police discourse on drug and alcohol-related violence might be regarded as dubious at best, given the not so distant cultural memory of NSW police praising New Year's Eve crowds in 2000 for their behaviour and attributing the lack of violent incidents to the widespread use of ecstasy (Bearup 2000). If a culture of peaceful nighttime sociability is the aim of police operations, it would appear they are happy to ignore their own corporate memory and intelligence in this instance.

While sniffer dogs have now become a staple feature of police responses to 'antisocial behaviour', their use was originally substantiated in relation to drug enforcement quite specifically. Drug dogs appeared in Sydney shortly after the Sydney 2000 Olympics and their use was formalised in the *Police Powers (Drug Detection Dogs) Act* (2001) after a court ruling challenged their legality. This form of policing can be understood as a form of 'show-policing': one of the first operations involved 300 police officers and the media units of all the major newspapers raiding a straight nightclub on Oxford Street, leading to the arrest of only two people. The effectiveness of the strategy has been thoroughly debunked in a review of the legislation conducted by the NSW Ombudsman (2006).[3] The practice appears to be driven more by the state's desire to be *seen to be doing something* than any serious attempt to address any problem associated with drugs. As a policing strategy, it stages an intense but ultimately superficial battle between the amoral market and the 'moral' state in an exercise of power I have termed 'exemplary power' (Race 2009). Without doubt, the strategy disproportionately affects those forms of urban culture that have been elaborated around the use of illicit drugs. As one letter-writer to the *Sydney Star Observer* put it recently: 'Understandably things change, but for a gay scene to have been almost obliterated is puzzling' (Marcus 2009). Just as distressing, the practice has led to a significant deterioration of relations built up carefully over many years between sexual minorities and the police. Over the past decade, drug policing performatively enacts NSW police as aggressive and homophobic – if not in intention, then certainly in effect.

Locked in by the lockout

This chapter is based on material I first pulled together in 2011. Since that time the situation it describes has only intensified. NSW drug dog operations have been scaled up over the last few years, and now feature as a regular and imposing presence at mainstream music festivals, dance parties, clubs, bars and recreational precincts. Meanwhile, relations between NSW police and sexual and gender minorities are at an all-time low. The increasingly heavy-handed policing of Mardi Gras, which has included documented instances of police brutality during the parade and aggressive drug dog operations at queer dance parties, galvanized thousands to participate in a large protest rally against police brutality and aggression the week after Mardi Gras, 2013. In 2014, a moral panic over nighttime violence in Kings Cross (a mainly heterosexual drinking scene these days) led the state government to impose licensing restrictions throughout the inner city, including Oxford Street, locking patrons out of all nighttime venues in the lockout zone from 1am. The effect has been to eradicate most visible signs of nightlife and dance culture in the inner city entirely, precipitating a further spate of massive public rallies and protests over 2016 (Race 2016). Needless to say, LGBTIQ subcultural participants have been particularly adversely affected by these governmental assaults, which have eradicated key spaces of socialisation for these communities, and driven gay partying underground.

I will return to this problem in the second part of this book when I examine the emergence of new spaces and practices of sexualised drug use. This chapter has demonstrated how drug practices have participated in the materialisation of urban gay culture historically. Sometimes drug use has served to excuse the self from regimes of heteronormativity and stigmatised sex, but it has also been valued for how it can transform the mood, atmosphere and vibe of communal infrastructures of sexual sociability and how the world feels to participants in these spaces and events. In addition to the significant role they have played in the formation and renewal of queer social bonds, parties have given rise to significant collective innovations in care practice. Obviously, drug practices are not the only practices through which gay community has been historically elaborated, and it remains to be seen whether they will continue to play such a significant role in the constitutive practices of urban gay culture given its diversification and integration into mainstream culture in recent years. But it would be difficult to understand the materialisation of urban gay identity without accounting for the cultural and historical activity of drugs.

Over the last century, the social consumption of intoxicating substances has been a key target of disciplinary attempts to privatise and normalise sexuality. But where previously police intervention targeted deviant expressions of sexuality and gender explicitly, in the post-liberation context it would appear that LGBTIQ social spaces have been ineptly or conveniently caught up in the government of nighttime violence and the nighttime economy, which nonetheless threatens these forms of sexual sociability. Public panic over nighttime violence and antisocial behaviour has generated a desire on the part of the state to be *seen to be doing something* in the highly mediatised environment of contemporary law and order, and this has led to the adoption of strategies of surveillance, intimidation and closure that are not only ill-fitted to the problem at hand, but disproportionately affect these forms of urban culture.

These interventions can be situated as part of ongoing disciplinary efforts to eradicate forms of public sociability that do not organise themselves around either the family or legitimate consumer markets. Given the historical use of dance drugs to elaborate its particular modes of urban belonging, it is not surprising that gay community has become the locus of some of the most vocal objections to this policing strategy. But while this strategy disproportionately affects queer and gay urban space, and is prone to homophobic abuse, a successful counter-response need not rest on the argument that these interventions unfairly target a minority identity exclusively. Rather, it can be grounded in the innovative and effective practices of social care and government associated with queer responses to HIV and drug harm, which have emphasised pleasure, care and cooperation rather than fear, intimidation and demonisation. On this basis, the care practices that make up good party practices may well achieve an exemplary power of their own.

Notes

1 RAT parties were dance parties hosted by the Recreational Arts Team, a group of artists and friends who used creative design concepts to throw extravagant, wildly popular dance parties throughout the 1980s in Sydney which attracted an inner-city crowd of heterosexual bohemians as well as gay men, lesbians and drag queens.

2 A number of high-profile police operations targeting 'drug and alcohol associated violence and anti-social behavior' were conducted throughout Sydney over the summers of 2007 and 2008, while licensing restrictions were imposed on a number of late-night venues in 2008. Even when the possibility of homophobic violence was raised, this generally translated into a call for 'more police'.

3 The review found that the strategy yielded trafficable quantities of drugs in only the tiniest percentage of indicated searches while three out of four searches failed to yield any illicit substances at all. Meanwhile, the strategy was found to generate even riskier practices of consumption as users attempted to avoid detection. See Race 2014.

References

Adam, B. 1987. *The Rise of a Gay and Lesbian Movement*. Boston: Twayne Publishers.
Ballard, J. 1992. Australia: Participation and innovation in a federal system. In D. Kirp & R. Bayer (eds.) *AIDS in Industrialized Democracies: Passions, Politics and Policies*. New Jersey: Rutgers University Press, pp. 134–167.
Bardella, C. 2002. Pilgrimages of the plagued: AIDS, body and society. *Body & Society*, 8(2), pp. 79–105.
Bearup, G. 4 January 2000. Love's in the air, alcohol nowhere. *Sydney Morning Herald*, p. 4.
Bech, H. 1997. *When Men Meet: Homosexuality and Modernity*. Chicago: University of Chicago Press.
Bell, D. & Binnie, J. 2000. *The Sexual Citizen*. Cambridge: Polity.
Bell, D. & Binnie, J. 2004. Authenticating queer space: Citizenship, urbanism and governance. *Urban Studies*, 41(9), pp. 1807–1820.
Berlant, L. & Warner, M. 1998. Sex in public. *Critical Inquiry*, 24(2), pp. 547–566.
Burn, C. 1 April 2009. Time to work together. *SX News* [online]. Retrieved from http://sxnews.gaynewsnetwork.com.au/feature/we-are-not-the-enemy-005219.html [4 June 2011].
Carbery, G. 1995. *A History of the Gay and Lesbian Mardi Gras*. Parkville: Australian Gay and Lesbian Archives.
Carter, D. 2004. *Stonewall: The riots that sparked the gay revolution*. New York: St. Martin's Press.
Chauncey, G. 1994. *Gay New York: Gender, urban culture, and the making of the gay male world 1890–1940*. New York: Basic Books.
Crowley, M. 1969. *The Boys in the Band*. London: Secker & Warburg.
Delany, S. 1999. *Times Square Red, Times Square Blue*. New York: New York University Press.
D'Emilio, J. 1983. *Sexual Politics, Sexual Communities*. Chicago: University of Chicago Press.
Duberman, M. 1993. *Stonewall*. London: Penguin Books.
Eribon, D. 2004. *Insult and the Making of the Gay Self*. Durham: Duke University Press.
Faro, C. 2000. *Street Seen: A History of Oxford St*. Melbourne: Melbourne University Press.
Ford, C. & Tyler, P. 1933. *The Young and Evil*. Paris: Obelisk Press.
Gibson, C. & Connell, J. 2000. Artistic dreamings: Tinseltown, Sin City and suburban wasteland. In J. Connell (ed.) *Sydney: The Emergence of a World City*. Oxford: Oxford University Press, pp. 292–318.

Gomart, E. & Hennion, A. 1998. A sociology of attachment: Music amateurs, drug users. *The Sociological Review*, 46(S), pp. 220–247.

Gonçalves, D., Kolstee, J., Ryan, D. & Race, K. 2016. Harm reduction in process: The ACON Rovers, GHB, and the art of paying attention. *Contemporary Drug Problems*, 43(4), pp. 314–330.

Green, A. 2003. 'Chem friendly': The institutional basis of club-drug use in a sample of urban gay men. *Deviant Behavior*, 24(5), pp. 427–447.

Guthmann, E. 15 January 1999. 70s gay film has low self esteem. *The San Francisco Chronicle* [online]. Retrieved from http://www.sfgate.com/movies/article/70s-Gay-Film-Has-Low-Esteem-Boys-attitude-2952305.php [21 January 2017].

Haire, B. 2001. Mardi Gras. In C. Johnston & P. Van Reyk (eds.) *Queer City: Gay and Lesbian Politics in Sydney*. Sydney: Pluto Press, pp. 97–111.

Halkitis, P., Parsons, J. & Stirratt, M. 2001. A double epidemic: Crystal methamphetamine drug use in relation to HIV transmission among gay men. *Journal of Homosexuality*, 41 (2), pp. 17–35.

Harvey, S. 2000. *The Ghost of Ludwig Gertsch*. Sydney: Pan Macmillan.

Hobbs, D., Hadfield, P., Lister, S., & Winlow, S. 2003. *Bouncers: Violence and Governance in the Night-Time Economy*. Oxford: Oxford University Press.

Holleran, A. 1978. *Dancer from the Dance*. London: Penguin.

Hurley, M. 2001. Sydney. In C. Johnston & P. Van Reyk (eds.) *Queer City: Gay and Lesbian Politics in Sydney*. Sydney: Pluto Press, pp. 241–257.

Lewis, L. & Ross, A. 1995. *A Select Body: The Gay Dance Party Culture and the HIV/ AIDS Pandemic*. New York: Cassell.

Malins, P. 2004. Machinic assemblages: Deleuze, Guattari and an ethico-aesthetics of drug use. *Janus Head*, 7(1), pp. 84–104.

Marcus. 20 October 2009. Memorial plaque. *Sydney Star Observer* [online]. Retrieved from http://www.starobserver.com.au/news/2009/10/20/letters-6/17412 [4 June 2011].

Markwell, K. 2002. Mardi Gras tourism and the construction of Sydney as an international gay and lesbian city. *GLQ*, 8(1–2), pp. 81–99.

Marsh, I. & Galbraith, L. 1995. The political impact of the Sydney gay and lesbian Mardi Gras. *Australian Journal of Political Science*, 30(2), pp. 300–320.

Masters, J. 2007. 'We promised never to tell!!' Confusions from the medical tent. Paper presented at *Queer Space: Centres and Peripheries*, University of Technology Sydney, Sydney, 20–1 February.

McKirnan, D., Ostrow, D. & Hope, B. 1996. Sex, drugs and escape: A psychological model of HIV-risk sexual behaviours. *AIDS Care*, 8(6), pp. 655–670.

McLachlan, M. 13 October 2009. Serious threat. *Sydney Star Observer* [online]. Retrieved from http://www.starobserver.com.au/news/2009/10/13/letters-to-the-editor-56/17098 [4 June 2011].

Muñoz, J. 2009. *Cruising Utopia*. New York: New York University Press.

NSW Ombudsman. 2006. *Review of the Police Powers (Drug Detection Dogs) Act 2001*. Sydney: NSW Government.

Quilley, S. 1997. Constructing Manchester's "New Urban Village": Gay space in the entrepreneurial city. In G. Ingram, A. Bouthillette & Y. Retter (eds.) *Queers in Space: Communities, Public Places, Sites of Resistance.* Washington: Bay Press, pp. 275–294.

Race, K. 2009. *Pleasure Consuming Medicine.* Durham: Duke University Press.

Race, K. 2014. Complex events: Drug effects and emergent causality. *Contemporary Drug Problems*, 41(3), pp. 301–334.

Race, K. 2016. The sexuality of the night: Violence and transformation. *Current Issues in Criminal Justice*, 28(1) pp. 105–110.

Sant, K. 18 March 2009. Step back in time. *SX News.* Retrieved from http://sxnews.gaynewsnetwork.com.au/feature/step-back-in-time-005133.html [4 June 2011].

Sendziuk, P. 2003. *Learning to Trust: Australian Responses to HIV/AIDS.* Sydney: UNSW Press.

Southgate, E. & Hopwood, M. 1999. Mardi Gras says 'be drug free': Accounting for resistance, pleasure and the demand for illicit drugs. *Health*, 3(3), pp. 303–316.

Stall, R. & Wiley, J. 1988. A comparison of alcohol and drug use patterns of homosexual and heterosexual men: The San Francisco Men's Health Study. *Drug and Alcohol Dependence*, 22, pp. 63–73.

Tomsen, S. 2001. Queer and safe: Combating violence with gentrified sexual identities. In C. Johnston & P. Van Reyk, (eds.) *Queer City: Gay and Lesbian Politics in Sydney*. Sydney: Pluto Press, pp. 229–240.

Waitt, G. & Markwell, K. 2003. *Gay Tourism: Culture and Context.* Binghamton: Haworth Press.

Wotherspoon, G. 1991. *City of the Plain: History of a Gay Subculture.* Sydney: Hale & Iremonger.

Young, I. 1990. *Justice and the Politics of Difference.* Princeton: Princeton University Press.

3 Click here for HIV status

Sorting for sexual partners

If HIV prevention has always had to 'get into' spaces of intimacy, this has been achieved in various ways. Though often experienced or presented these days as an obstacle to intimacy, the condom was initially proposed within the urban gay subcultures that confronted the looming health crisis as a convenient solution to the problem of disease transmission and a means of *access* to intimacy. Here, intimacy was taken to stretch beyond the bounds of the conjugal couple, with sex operating not simply as a private exchange between familiar partners but as a mode of social participation capable of generating new relational possibilities and affective climates even among relative strangers: a sense of collective belonging, camaraderie, play and social enjoyment bearing exciting possibilities of self-transformation (Foucault 1997; Warner 2000). Some appreciation of the elasticity of intimacy and sex at least seems to have informed the initial proposal of 'safe sex' on the part of gay activists and queer community leaders, who largely rejected calls for abstinence, monogamy and mandatory testing and drew instead on available wisdom about how the disease was most likely to be transmitted and shared practical advice about how to avoid transmitting the disease among peers and strangers on this basis (Watney 1988; Patton 1990; Escoffier 1998; Kippax & Race 2003; Halperin 2007). This advice was specifically fitted to the cultures of casual sex that had become a feature of urban gay enclaves among other places over the course of the twentieth century, enacting these cultures as a constellation of ongoing practices that with some minor modification would enable participants to overcome the crisis.

In these early articulations of safe sex, the condom featured as one tool within flexible sexual repertoires that presented multiple possibilities for HIV prevention (Crimp 1987; Kippax et al. 1993). An explicit but often forgotten aim of these early codes of HIV prevention was to cultivate and sustain a 'poz-friendly' (HIV-positive) communal environment (Race 2003). It was believed those infected with the virus should not be precluded from participation in gay sex or the communal spaces associated with it, which were thought to offer crucial sustenance in this time of loss and crisis (see Figure 3.1). From this perspective, the collective modification of sexual practice through bodily experimentation and communal education was a much more promising, appealing and practical prospect than competing propositions, such as the medico-legal proposal to identify infected individuals through HIV testing and foreclose their participation in sexual culture (Sendziuk 2003; Kippax & Race 2003). The latter proposal was deemed not only impractical but also unnecessarily divisive, insofar as it would subject those identified as HIV-positive to sexual and social rejection and effectively exclude them from the sexual community. 'Treat everyone as though they might be positive and always use a condom' was the maxim that guided many participants through gay sexual settings over the crisis years, and this practical ethic had the benefit of ruling out the difficulties, awkwardness, sheer nerve and imposition of asking friends, strangers and people one has just met their HIV status.

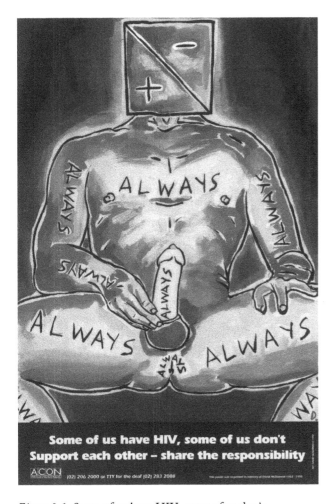

Figure 3.1 Some of us have HIV, some of us don't.

1990s ACON campaign featuring artwork by David McDiarmid, 1992. Courtesy of ACON

This positioning of the condom as an *enabling* (rather than restrictive) device does not necessarily make latex technology fun or easy or all that appealing to use, especially over the long term, and within the decade gay sexual subjects in Western locations began experimenting with other means of HIV prevention – practices that were more or less acknowledged, ignored, formalised or condemned by discourses of HIV prevention in different locations (Race 2003). I begin to explore the social and material effects of these different degrees of receptivity to gay men's experiments with HIV prevention in Chapter 4. Here I focus on one such innovation, now known as 'serosorting', which involves seeking out sexual partners of like HIV status to minimise the risks of penetrative sex, including sex that dispenses with condoms. I consider how the digital infrastructures of online cruising began to consolidate this practice within gay men's sexual repertoires at the turn of the millennium, and how these sexual infrastructures began to shape relations between users and their bodies in material ways to create new problems and possibilities for HIV prevention. While variable in format, online cruising sites mediate sexual partnering in quite specific ways that differ significantly from those characterising the settings within which men had become accustomed to hooking up for sex. In this chapter I ask: How did participants in this changing sexual culture first respond to this new sexual infrastructure? How did they learn to negotiate the modes of interaction and partner selection its mechanisms proposed, and with what effects? What impact did the introduction of this infrastructure have on the terms through which participants were being made (and making themselves) into subjects of HIV prevention?

An initial picture of this process can be gleaned from trends collected in the Sydney Gay Community Periodic Survey, a cross-sectional study conducted annually among homosexually active men (Zablotska et al. 2007). From 2000 onwards, these data reveal a substantial increase in the proportion of men who reported looking for sex online, and a shift away from more established settings for cruising such as bars, beats, sex venues and dance parties (see Figure 3.2). This increase is particularly apparent among HIV-negative and untested men. HIV-positive men emerge in these data as 'early adopters' of online platforms for sexual purposes, insofar as a higher proportion of them were using this medium to arrange sex from the first time data on this question was collected (see Figure 3.3). Alongside these trends, from 1998 onwards the proportion of respondents who reported disclosing their HIV status to some or all of their sexual partners increased significantly (see Figure 3.4), while the proportion of men who did not disclose their HIV status to any of their sexual partners began to drop. These trends reached a tipping point in 2002, with increasing HIV disclosure in sexual contexts evident among the Sydney men surveyed, irrespective of HIV status (see Figure 3.5). These data do not tell us where all this HIV disclosure was occurring (or for what purpose), but the parallels between these trends are striking. Evidently, disclosing HIV status to sexual partners increased in tandem with the increasing use of the Internet to arrange sex over this period. By 2004 the Internet had become the primary

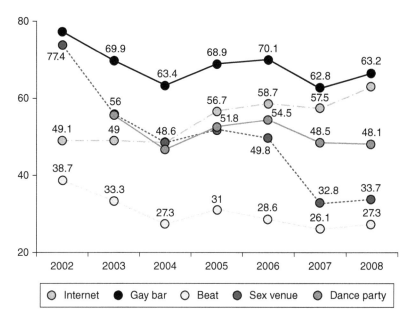

Figure 3.2 Where men looked for sexual partners.

Source: Zablotska et al. 2008

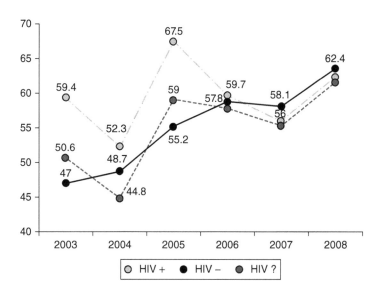

Figure 3.3 Men who looked for sex online, by serostatus.

Source: Zablotska et al. 2008

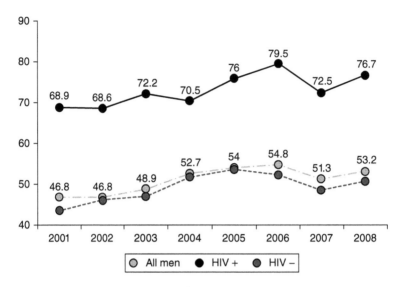

Figure 3.4 Proportion of men who disclosed their HIV status to some or all sexual partners.

Source: Zablotska et al. 2008

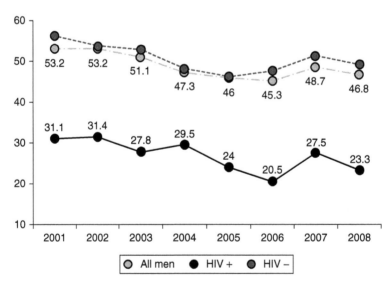

Figure 3.5 Proportion of men who did not disclose their HIV status to any sexual partners.

Source: Zablotska et al. 2008

venue in or through which Sydney gay men looked for sex, alongside bars. While it is unclear from these data whether these men necessarily 'got' what they were looking for online, the growing popularity of digitally arranged sex corresponds chronologically with documented increases in what might safely be assumed to be attempted serosorting.

These increases in HIV-negative disclosure for casual sex became a source of particular concern in Australia. While HIV-positive disclosure tends to be supported, even by more conservative HIV prevention authorities (which sometimes mandate it), disclosing an HIV-negative status to unknown sexual partners as a way of reducing risk is an entirely different prospect. When operating as a basis for dispensing with condoms during casual sex, it can be viewed as problematic on a number of grounds – not least, the possibility that sexual partners may not know (or may lie) about their status. The problem is further complicated by the technical limitations perceived in the standard tests used to detect HIV infection in clinical practice at this time – specifically, their ability to detect the presence of the HIV virus *in vivo*. It was possible to be infected with HIV but show up as 'HIV-negative' according to these antibody tests, because the development of antibodies in the bodies of infected individuals takes place sometime after infection with the virus ('the window period') – which could be up to two or three months, going on medical opinion of the time. Given what is also known about the immune system response and the dynamics of viral replication in the context of initial infection, this stage is widely thought to be when a body is most infectious. Thus, when serosorting was first discussed in Australia, an HIV-negative test result was not considered a reliable guide to whether a body was infected (or, for that matter, infectious). Indeed, in the context of recent episodes of potential exposure to the virus (which might well be repeat episodes if the presenting individual has been attempting to sort for HIV-negative casual partners), the standard HIV antibody test could just as easily function as precisely the opposite: an unreliable intermediary with potentially dangerous consequences.

Given these concerns and contingencies, I want to use this opportunity to think about how the growing immersion in online cruising at this time was beginning to shape sexual and risk subjectivities. Online cruising sites lend themselves to particular practices of sexual socialising and casual partnering which bear the potential to inform general repertoires of HIV prevention in sexual contexts. How were gay men negotiating the tensions between competing practices of attempted HIV prevention that began to circulate at this time – specifically, those that operationalise HIV status as a precursor to sex and those that didn't? Elsewhere, I have explored how the uptake of antiretroviral therapy and its clinical devices generated changes in some men's sexual and risk practices (Race 2001, 2003). Here, I am interested in how the new interfaces of digital sex began to mediate investments in HIV disclosure as a prelude to sexual sociability.

As well as installing new criteria for partner selection, I am interested in how these mechanisms participate in the emergence of particular affective climates and contours of experience, which in turn give rise to different practical possibilities (and indeed impossibilities) for differently situated sexual actors. To develop the idea of affective climates, I draw on Latour's suggestion that sociotechnical assemblages are composed of 'bodies learning to be affected by hitherto unregistrable differences through the mediation of an artificially created set-up' (Latour 2004, p. 209). This conception is appealing because it conceives of bodies as always enmeshed within socio-technical arrangements, with nothing presumed about the nature of humans or their psychological states. It directs attention to the specificities of the technical arrangements within which bodies come into contact, apprehend and impact one another. Bodies are always enmeshed within specific structures of entanglement, which make certain capacities, relations and powers of acting available. Investigating how particular affective climates are mediated and co-produced may afford some insight into the changing contours and conditions within which people conduct their sex lives (among other everyday practices). I want to understand how participants in these new sexual infrastructures – which included people of different HIV statuses, among other social categories – accounted for, managed and made use of the affordances they perceived in them.

Before the introduction of smartphone apps in 2009, *Gaydar* and *Manhunt* were the most popular gay cruising sites in Sydney with each attracting an average of about 1,000 active users on a given Friday or Saturday night. This chapter draws on observations made while using these sites, which I extend by drawing on qualitative interviews with Sydney gay men (n = 31) conducted as part of a study in 2006–7. A particular focus of the enquiry was HIV-negative men's feelings and perceptions of the presence of HIV-positive individuals in the sexual environments they shared with them. From the late 1990s, increasing emphasis was placed internationally on the responsibilities of HIV-positive individuals for HIV prevention, reflected in increasing prosecutions of HIV-positive people for transmission offences around the world (Race 2001; Hoppe 2017). We were aware that a number of practical obstacles impede disclosure of HIV status on the part of HIV-positive individuals in casual settings, including not wanting to disclose sensitive health information, fear of rejection and gossip, and the general lack of verbal communication that characterises many of the relevant venues such as saunas. Concerned that a proportion of HIV-negative men might be operating under the false impression that HIV-positive men routinely announce their HIV status before sex, we wanted to explore HIV-negative men's assumptions about the sexual fields in which they participated, their thoughts about the prospect of sero-discordant sex, and their predisposition towards HIV-positive participants. Another concern was how HIV-positive participants were being affected by social technologies that increasingly held them responsible for HIV transmission and its prevention.

From cruising to browsing

In many ways, online cruising is analogous to other practices of sexual socialising already familiar to gay men in that it brings certain aspects of consumer
subjectivity to bear on sexual relations. In her discussion of the design of gay
bathhouses or saunas, Dianne Chisolm illustrates how these venues sexualised
the logic of the shopping arcade, for example (Chisolm 2005, pp. 10–17).
Similar logics became evident when we spoke to gay men about the attraction
of online cruising sites.

> Sean: [On cruising online] It's great in terms of accessibility 24/7. I can
> organise my sex around my work schedule. It's also like a shopping cart.
> You can go, 'Okay, I'm interested in Caucasian men', or whatever, down
> to sexual preference. It's about being able to access an immediate selec-
> tion of people you might be interested in. I think that is a bonus.
>
> (Thirty-four years old, 2007)

Since online cruising sites are generally designed and used with the aim
of constructing offline erotic relations, it would be wrong to characterise
them in terms of a radical rupture with offline sexual contexts and practices
(Hardey 2002). Rather, use of the Internet is threaded through urban gay
sexual culture, supporting, extending, reconfiguring and interfering with
existing venues of sexual socialising while drawing on many of their genres
and conventions to devise specific forms of functionality. As online cruising
sites became more popular, it became common for people to point out others according to their online profile names in bars and clubs, as though this
were another titbit of information that rounded out someone's personality.
Meanwhile, at social venues, people started to give out their profile name
instead of hooking up immediately – a practice that extends the temporality
of sexual availability (sometimes indefinitely!) while displacing 'picking up'
as the predominant modus operandi of the gay 'night out'. In early cyber-
studies, much was made of the possibility of transcending the constraints of
space and gender identity in virtual space (Van Zoonen 2002), but the connection between online activity and offline objectives in the case of online
cruising sites indicates the need to qualify such claims. Profiles are typically organised into rooms in a given location and online interaction takes
place on the implicit understanding that participants are accessible in that
location – if not now, then at some time in the future. Moreover, if too
great a difference becomes apparent between a user's online persona and their
'real-life' identity or appearance, this is seen by other users as deception or
fraudulence, and commonly provokes disappointment, contempt, ridicule or
at best uneasy compromise.

The main mode of online participation on cruising sites is 'browsing', in which
users inspect webpages and conduct searches according to their preferences.

Various methods exist to signal interest and further communication, such as sending winks, making use of various messaging options and exchanging or revealing private pictures with other users. The central mechanism of these websites is the online profile, in which users deploy the formatting options available to frame their personal appearance and interests. On many gay cruising sites, online profiles are composed of a mix of public and private photos ('pics') and users are variously presented with the option to share private pics with other users of their choice. There is generally space for open-ended description of oneself on the profile page, which is populated predominantly by pro-forma items that offer categories via drop-down menus according to which users can specify personal attributes and interests.

Mark Davis and colleagues have usefully characterised one of the key modes of online participation as 'filtering' (Davis et al. 2006). As they discuss, the Internet allows the 'quiet sorting' of partners via the images and texts that depict and construct sexual personae. Online cruising is distinctive in that it allows users to stage their online presence to their own advantage, gradually releasing information about their appearance, attributes and interests to potential partners. Users 'market' themselves on their profiles according to their perceptions of others' desires and their own decisions about how best to position themselves within the sexual marketplace to get what they want (or what they can). In this regard, the online profile can be conceived as a 'market device' (Callon et al. 2007) that equips users with certain capacities and formats practices of self-representation, informing activities such as searching, evaluating, sorting and selecting among the various 'goods' on offer.

The opportunity to state and view sexual preferences on public profiles concretises a field of sexual value which elevates expressions of sexual preference to broadcast status. For example:

> Only interested in guys under 30.
>
> No fats, fems, or Asians
>
> Drug and Disease Free, UB2

In being given textual expression, the selective and exclusionary character of people's sexual preferences took on a new materiality. Little wonder that the growing immersion in online cruising generated a sharp critique of 'sexual racism' within gay community discourse (Mansfield & Quan 2006). While prejudice against certain racialised minorities has long been a documented feature of Australian gay culture (Ayres 1999; Han 2006), rarely had such prejudice been so explicit and routinely visible, with race/ethnicity featuring not only as an inbuilt category of identification but also expressly and voluntarily embedded into the textual landscape of sexual preferences that gay men found themselves having to navigate in their attempts to connect with others. There is always some scope for critical and creative intervention in such situations. For example, when constructing their online profiles participants sometimes use whatever open response options might be available to criticise annoying statements or objectionable gestures they commonly encounter when using these media. For example:

> Ignorant people who repel people on this website based on race, don't bother to contact me.

> I don't respond to winks, it's not that hard boys to string a few words together.

> Send me winks, I think they're great little flirts, what's the worst that can happen?

But while there are certain opportunities to construct one's online presence in a way that critically intervenes in the criteria of value that constitute these sexual fields, members' profiles are largely populated by mandatory categories of self-description with limited response options. The significance of this can be seen if we consider how HIV prevention preferences were formatted on Gaydar.com and Manhunt.net at this time.

Gaydar was founded in November 1999 by the UK-based company QSoft Consulting and became the most popular gay cruising site in Sydney shortly thereafter.[1] Early versions of the website offered a number of profile categories according to which users could specify their attributes ranging from their physical appearance and sexual preferences to their hobbies, favourite movies, pastimes and leisure interests. Participants could indicate their preference for safer sex according to the following options: 'Always', 'Sometimes', 'Never', 'Needs Discussion' and 'Rather Not Say' – and could choose whether to display or hide this item on their profile. While it was technically possible to disclose one's HIV status in the open-ended sections of the profile, few users revealed such information at the time of analysis, and no prompts around HIV status existed on the website.

Compare Manhunt, established by the US-based company Online Buddies Inc. in 2001, which went on to become the most popular gay cruising site in Sydney over the next decade.[2] Manhunt featured a faster and sexier temporality than its competitors, mainly by virtue of its 'unlock' feature, which allowed users to unlock their private photos for other users without further communication in one stroke of the keyboard. Its profile categories are largely organised around sexual interests (no hobbies or movie dates on offer here): thus the site addresses itself to, and constitutes, a 'racier' sexual market. With regard to HIV prevention preferences, if the British proponents of Gaydar would 'Rather Not Say', the US producers and consumers of Manhunt seem much more invested in self-disclosure as a highway to truth and safety. At the time of analysis, the site required users to specify their HIV status directly using the options it made available: 'Ask me', 'Negative', 'Positive', 'Unknown' and 'No Answer'. There was no mechanism for users to hide this item on their profile – thus selecting 'No Answer' would appear on one's profile as

'HIV STATUS: [blank]'. In other words, even when left unanswered, the question on HIV status took the form of a compulsory prompt on this platform. In terms of the impact of this development, the founding date of Manhunt is significant. If we consider the trends depicted in Figure 3.3 we can see that a marked increase in HIV status disclosure on the part of Sydney gay men corresponds with the 2001 introduction of Manhunt. As far as I can determine, this was the first sexual environment that routinely asked Sydney gay men to indicate their HIV status as *a design feature of participation*.

How users of these sites deploy and interpret the identifiers that constitute the online profile is, of course, another significant question. Davis and colleagues document some reluctance on the part of the British HIV-positive men they interviewed to list their HIV status explicitly: this was seen as embarrassing, tactless and a detail that would most likely jar with the affective flows and dynamics of cruising (Davis et al. 2006). Their sample of gay men tended to deal with concerns around HIV prevention primarily by indicating their preferences around safe sex. Thus some HIV-positive Gaydar users in London reported signalling their HIV status by selecting options other than 'Safer sex: Always' – the most common specification on Gaydar profiles at the time. In addition, HIV-negative participants tended to read this as an indication of HIV-positive status – or at least a risky proposition.

These findings were mirrored in the accounts given by participants in our 2006 study. The HIV-positive men we interviewed generally regarded the Internet as a space in which they could signal their HIV status to other men without always having explicitly to disclose it.

> Ray: I have put whatever the appropriate option is. Some [websites] don't have positive as an option. They say 'barebacking' but I don't necessarily choose that as an option. I will choose 'after discussion' or something; that is usually the option I have to choose. But if you hook up over the Internet it's not guaranteed that someone will disclose – you can't guarantee it.
>
> (HIV-positive, forty-seven years old, 2007)

> Interviewer: You don't have it on your profile?
> Chahaya: In a way I do. There's a category which says 'safe sex' and I say 'needs discussion' which really means I'm HIV-positive more or less. Although some people don't get it, as though it's a little bit obtuse.
>
> (HIV-positive, forty-six years old, 2008)

> Carl: If someone says on their website that they are into unprotected sex then I would not go with anyone who says they do that and I would specify that there is no negotiation on that. Generally I won't even reply if they put that on their website; I find it a real turn-off.
>
> (HIV-negative, thirty-five years old, 2007)

The interpretation and use of the HIV status prompt on Manhunt were less clear. In Sydney at this time, specification of HIV-negative status was by far the most common response to this profile prompt, while admission of HIV-positive status was relatively rare. But such tendencies varied geographically and regionally. In my own experience of using this site, I found HIV-positive disclosure to be much more common in San Francisco, New York and Sydney than it was in locations such as Ann Arbor, Hobart and Melbourne – each of which have smaller gay scenes without the same sort of critical mass of openly HIV-positive gay men and fewer opportunities for anonymity in gay circles. Despite this regional variation, we can see the potential of these websites to generate new norms and expectations around HIV disclosure and make new demands of sexual subjects. To quote from an HIV-negative user's Manhunt profile in Sydney, 2008:

> Be honest about your status, if no status listed then there will be no response.

Thus, while these self-identifiers operate according to different logics and constraints in different locations, the part they play in the construction of new norms and affective climates of sexual interaction is potentially quite significant.

So far I have discussed the emergence of a significant new sexual infrastructure that began to transform the terms and practices of gay sex and social interaction in urban gay centres in the first decade of the millennium. This infrastructure cannot be considered independent or entirely extricable from longer-standing venues and spaces of gay sexual sociability, insofar as use of it interweaves with participation in these contexts. We can nonetheless see how this digital infrastructure proposed new modes of sexual self-presentation, new ways of relating to prospective sexual partners and new investments in HIV disclosure, and made new experiences of convenience and avoidance possible. This medium elevated personal expressions of sexual preference to broadcast status, giving them a textual materiality that other users found themselves having to navigate. Participation was animated by a 'browser' subjectivity, in which prospective partners could be scanned for sexual compatibility according to a range of pre-defined criteria. Such calculations could be made on the basis of a range of texts, images and category markers: digital images of physical appearance and tick-a-box expressions of sexual preference and personal attributes primarily. These templates and formats of sexual partnering also became available to be carried over into other contexts, informing and interfering with practical logics of gay sexual interaction more generally, as I will go on to consider.

The problem with disclosure

A number of HIV-negative men we interviewed for this study declared some degree of adherence to well-established prevention ethics: assume any of your casual sexual partners might be HIV-positive and take appropriate precautions. This ethic was typically articulated in relation to the norms of non-disclosure that had characterised the operation of gay sex venues histori-cally. Among these men, the use of condoms tended to function as a practical substitute for asking or wanting to know their partners' HIV status. We found this to be the case even among many of the younger men we spoke with:

> Caleb: I have a thing about disclosure, because I think that it's unfair to expect someone to disclose when I know that it would be an issue. It must be so impossible to disclose, particularly in a casual situation. I don't think disclosure is a responsibility. It's a bonus. I just think everyone's potentially HIV-positive, that's how I deal with it.
>
> (Twenty-two years old, 2007)

> Interviewer: Do you have any preferences around the HIV status of people you have had sex with? And how do you find those partners if you have a preference?
> Adrian: Well I'm sure the preference, I would love everyone to be nega-tive, and just be like that, but I suppose the fact of the matter is that it's not really discussed. No one discloses – well I shouldn't generalise – but to me no one is disclosing and to be honest, I'm not disclosing to them, so I suppose that is the thing. It's not talked about.
> Interviewer: So how do you deal with that – what do you do to hopefully stay negative in those circumstances?
> Adrian: Condoms, condoms. And to be honest I don't really ask, and I don't know if it's I don't want to know, or if I – I've never really thought about that too much, but it's just not talked about, it's just not discussed.
>
> (Twenty-one years old, 2008)

These participants seem to have given some thought to the difficulties and challenges faced by HIV-positive participants in gay sexual cultures and ven-ues. Many of them were informed by a working knowledge of what might be realistically expected of HIV-positive strangers – what it is possible for them to say and do – in the context of the historical and practical constraints on sex between men in casual sex settings:

> Interviewer: Do you expect them to disclose?
> Daniel: Well, within the last twelve months I slept with someone who didn't and I found out through somebody else, which is fine, because I wasn't really so involved with that person, it was just sex. I can imagine that it is quite hard for a person to disclose regardless of their status. I'm sure that, because I have had casual sex before, and I might be in a backroom with someone playing around with somebody and for them to say, 'by the way before you get started, I'd like to tell you. . .' That is really unrealistic.
>
> (Twenty-six years old, 2007)

Interviewer: Who do you think should take the responsibility, the positive person or negative person or. . .?

Ralph: I think each person has to take their own responsibility and one person can't – well I say that, but I know how difficult it probably is to say . . . it's probably a lot easier to say, 'Hi I'm negative here, how about you?' So it's probably a lot more difficult for the positive person to say – especially if they have a desire and are attracted to this person, then they probably think, 'I really want this person, so I probably am only going to tell them what I think they want to hear'. Can be dangerous!

(Sixty-seven years old, 2007)

Tex: I think that sometimes there is an assumption that because this person has not said anything they are not poz. That is a big assumption.

(Thirty-four years old, 2007)

Participants had clearly engaged with the situation of HIV-positive participants in casual sex, apparently prompted by recent community education initiatives in some instances:

Interviewer: Have you thought that positive men might be a bit unkeen to tell people?

Ghazi: Yes, I read it as well, and I'm thinking, especially from my reaction, if I knew someone was positive I wouldn't go out with them, so I can understand that they don't want to get rejected, and I'm sure it's happened before to these guys as well, that's why they withhold it.

(Twenty-nine years old, 2007)

Interviewer: Do you have any preferences around the status of the people you have sex with and what motivates those preferences and how do you find partners of the same status, if that's what you do?

Caleb: I think everyone has a preference for safety. I don't really play into the serosorting – whatever they call it – like picking between positive and negative. I just sort of assume everyone is positive, I take safety precautions with everyone and then I try not to think about it, because if you do think about it there's always the window there for prejudices to come in and I don't really want to treat people on a prejudice base. The few times where it has come up I've continued to have sex with that person, but I can't say positively that that would be the experience in every situation. I think it depends on lots of things – how attracted I am, how into it I am, and maybe if I'm willing to take that risk in that particular situation. But to be honest I think my rules are for me to follow and I just make the assumption that everyone is positive and just don't think about it is sort of how I deal with it.

(Twenty-three years old, 2008)

Negative reactions to sero-discordant sex

When asked how they would react to a casual partner disclosing an HIV-positive status, HIV-negative men's reactions were mixed:

Interviewer: What would you do if they were positive?
Adonis: I wouldn't have any sexual relations with them. I wouldn't leave, I'd be prepared to talk to them or stay in bed with them, but that's really it.

(Twenty-six years old, 2008)

Ron: If they disclosed that they were positive to me? Well if someone says that to me, firstly I am sort of thankful that they have, it's a sign of intimacy really that they disclose to you, and so I take that as a very positive thing, affirming thing. Of course it's a clear indication – I guess the subtext is that we must use condoms, and so it's actually – to me, I have no concerns having sex with someone HIV-positive with condoms, and being careful, that is not a concern for me.

(Forty-eight years old, 2008)

Toby: I have been presented with – I've actually asked guys that I'm about to go with about their status – and sometimes some of them have said 'yes, I'm positive' and I've said 'thanks for telling me' and I haven't stopped. Obviously I have provided protection, but I can understand that there must be a lot of rejection, and for that reason I think that they would just rather not talk about it, and as long – like I say there is very little conversation in the sauna – so, as long as a condom is being introduced, then there is no real reason to have the conversation in the first place.

(Thirty-seven years old, 2007)

Interestingly, the 'poz-friendly' attitude Toby articulates above is expressly conditioned by his experience of live sex venues such as saunas, where condoms have emerged as the most convenient way of handling the potential risks of the situation. This construction of condoms as a substitute for having to know the HIV status of one's sexual contacts was not uncommon among the HIV-negative men in this sample. Indeed for some, the prospect of having sex with a partner known to be HIV-positive provoked a degree of anxiety that was so uncomfortable for them that they generally avoided actively seeking out such foreknowledge:

Interviewer: So if someone disclosed upfront, would you still have sex with them if it was safe and whatever?
Ghazi: No, no. Because I think that while we are having sex, that thing would be constantly on my mind, and so I wouldn't be able to perform, and then even maybe after the performance I would be worried that

something might have happened. But I don't go asking guys 'are you positive or not?' So, if one time I met someone and brought them home or I went to their place and then had sex with them and later on found out, then yeah. But I don't go asking whether they *are* or not.

(Thirty-one years old, 2008)

One can only speculate how the introduction of digital sorting capabilities might alter how this predisposition manifests in practical terms. Presumably, an open indication of HIV-positive status on someone's online profile would tip the balance for Ghazi and rule that person out as a prospective sexual partner, irrespective of the protection condoms offer.

Serosorting: from prevention to avoidance

While condoms balanced the need to know their partners' HIV status for many participants with some experience of face-to-face sex venues, at this time HIV-negative men were also becoming familiar with the possibilities of sorting newly afforded by digital interfaces. We can see how the templates and formats of online cruising serve to establish conditions for new investments in HIV status disclosure in the following accounts:

Interviewer: Are there any ways that guide the way you try and screen for negative people generally?
Baden: No, no. I guess the only way I would screen is if I was looking through some profiles on an Internet site, if someone admitted they were positive, I probably wouldn't pursue that, which is probably a bit hypocritical really, but I suppose I'm just not trying to court the risk I assume. I admire them, I really admire those guys who come out and say straight up 'you need to know this' because I think they are the people that we should be looking up to – but I don't feel like I need to add myself to that group, you know.

(Forty-four years old, 2008)

Interviewer: Do you expect positive people to always disclose?
Carl: Stupidly yes, I do actually. Or, if I was to ask, I would expect some honesty – and I've always asked. I wouldn't ask someone I'm having safe sex with, but I *have* asked people who I haven't had safe sex with – like, beforehand. And I assume they're telling the truth. It's stupid I know, these people don't need to protect me, they don't know you, they don't owe you anything.

(Thirty-five years old, 2007)

From Carl's account, it is possible to imagine how automated HIV disclosure might begin to play a more instrumental role in the potential arrangement of unprotected sex, tipping the balance between using condoms and assuming/avoiding.

Affective complications

Given the assumptions our research team held when embarking on this study, we found the reflexive processes many of our HIV-negative participants were clearly engaging in encouraging. These accounts gave insights into how these men were negotiating the tensions between the collective prevention ethics first elaborated in offline sexual contexts and the possibilities of filtering and sorting newly afforded by online formats. There was little evidence of attitudinal prejudice on the part of HIV-negative men in these data (which is not to say such prejudice did not exist in Sydney's gay cultures of the time).[3] Rather, what seemed to be apparent were a range of concerns, anxieties and makeshift solutions to the problem of self-protection, some of which are captured in the process of transformation in response to their cumulative encounters with the affordances of digital cruising. Where previously HIV-negative men were encouraged to presume all their sexual partners were HIV-positive and modify their sexual practice accordingly, these findings reveal a more complex mix of presumptions and practices, including underlying anxieties, concerns and in some instances a degree of wishful thinking that casual partners were most likely HIV-negative unless circumstances (such as a reluctance to disclose HIV status) indicated otherwise. If condoms 'solved' the problem of HIV transmission for many gay men historically by enabling them to ignore the question of their partners' HIV status, these data suggest that, even in the presence of condoms, knowledge that a partner is HIV-positive may provoke significant anxiety and avoidance for some HIV-negative people. The introduction of automated indications of HIV status on online profiles played an active part in transforming the associative patterns of gay sex. Online cruising templates contributed to the emergence of a new state of 'seronormativity' within these spaces at this time, transforming presumptions about the default HIV status of prospective sexual partners while placing new premiums on HIV status disclosure.

The increasing pressure on HIV-positive participants to disclose their status complicated their participation in gay sexual culture. While many HIV-positive gay men appreciated the digital capacity to find partners of like HIV status, the entextualisation of HIV status as a prelude to further communication – indeed, its encoding as a compulsory prompt and design feature of participation on some platforms – reconfigured the sexual marketplace in ways that many found frustrating and depressing. To give some sense of the dilemmas this changing landscape posed for HIV-positive participants, and the sorts of reactions and responses it provoked, some HIV-positive men's responses to this situation are assembled below:

> Darcy: I talk about my status and if that freaks them out, then that freaks them out. You get used to being rejected because of that, and well, so what? It's that sort of thing. But I'm not going to allow that to upset me, because I feel that if I'm being honest with them, I'm doing what I can to protect myself and them.
>
> (Seventy-one years old, 2007)

Ray: I'm getting to the point where the whole negotiating thing around my health status, I am agonising over it. Legally I'm supposed to tell them. Sometimes you never even exchange a word, so how do you tell them?

(Forty-seven years old, 2007)

Karl: Well, when I first was diagnosed, I wasn't interested in sex I suppose, but when I started having sex again, I found that I couldn't actually get an erection unless I told the partner. At the same time I was thinking, as far as casual sex goes, you meet someone once, and never see them again, and so trying to tell them something personal, when I haven't told some of my family members . . . I found that pretty weird. Now that I'm undetectable [i.e. viral levels are suppressed by treatment] I don't feel any responsibility to tell a partner, because I don't think there is any danger of passing it on. I don't want to tell them something personal that they might go and tell someone else.

(Forty-six years old, 2007)

Baxter: I think negative people, umm [pause]. I have had the experience where someone has wanted to have unsafe sex, and I disclose my status, and then they've rejected me because they didn't think I was positive, so there is that, and . . . you know, it's humiliating. And at the same time you feel like telling them, 'get a life'. And the whole undercurrent that comes with it. It's not a very nice feeling to say 'you are the baddie in the book'. And so, anyway. . .

(Forty-six years old, 2007)

Henry: I have found the community is quite divided. Some people are very ignorant, in particular about HIV and what it does to you and how you can catch it. There is still stigma attached to it. I can't disclose to everybody. It would just complicate my life too much.

(Forty-six years old, 2008)

As is evident in these accounts, the concretisation of HIV disclosure as a normative expectation in everyday sexual contexts had become a source of disaffection among HIV-positive gay men. This was compounded by gay men's increasingly common encounters with online cruising formats and mechanisms over this period. Indeed, among the accounts above, only Darcy reports successful adherence to a policy of disclosing his status to all his sexual partners, at the age of seventy-one. On his own account this requires of him an uncommonly blasé attitude towards the likelihood of sexual rejection.

The prospect of having to disclose their HIV status to new acquaintances and random strangers in sexual contexts is experienced by most of these men as a vexing problem. But the sort of problem it was, and the solutions that different individuals propose or tried to experiment with in response to it, depended on how they problematised the situation they found themselves experiencing, and 'the practices on the basis of which these problematizations were formed' (Foucault 1990, p. 11). Among the concerns and practices voiced above, we see a number of intelligible apprehensions: not wanting to confront rejection and humiliation from guys one finds sexually interesting; not wanting to disclose sensitive and personal health information to casual acquaintances; and the (potentially well-founded) presumption that others might treat them contemptuously, judge or demonise them for being HIV-positive. Meanwhile, the tendency *not* to disclose one's HIV status was rationalised on various grounds: the (non)-communicative conditions that operated in the contexts in which they usually hooked up; the presence of condoms; and speculation that effective suppression of viral load through the use of antiretroviral therapy ruled out the possibility of passing on the virus.

Though constrained by similar apprehensions and shared social circumstances, the solutions discussed above generally take the form of personal decisions. As Foucault argued, there are always several possible ways of responding to 'the same ensemble of difficulties' (Ong and Collier 2005, p. 43). Some of these are individualised, while other responses institute new collectives and infrastructures. An example of the latter is the website referenced earlier, *Sexual Racism Sux* (Mansfield & Quan 2006), which took the rejection, rudeness and exclusion commonly experienced by non-Anglo men online to constitute a particular sort of problem ('sexual racism') that demanded some sort of response – in this instance, the attempted activation of a critical public by setting up a website and online forum on the topic. Another collective response, in this case to HIV-positive disaffection with the sexual marketplace as it was being enacted by mainstream gay websites at this time, was the creation in 2004 of BarebackRealTime (BBRT), an online cruising site that set out to enable its members (presumed mainly to be HIV-positive) to cruise for hookups safely without confronting the sort of hostility they commonly experienced on 'gay-stream' sites like Manhunt. As I will discuss in Chapter 4, BBRT effectively flipped the terms of seronormativity by alternatively technologising the bodies and subjectivities of its members.

Biosociality and digital sex

Nikolas Rose and Carlos Novas have used the term 'digital bio-citizenship' to describe practices of prudence and responsibility in which individuals draw on medical knowledge and digital technologies to act upon and manage the implications of their corporeal being (2005, p. 442). Such regimes of self-management are implicit in the design of online dating sites such as positivesingles.com and safesexpassport.com, where individuals with (or without) sexually transmitted infections seek similarly infected (or uninfected) partners. To some extent, similar practices of prudence and selectivity have emerged as a characteristic feature of dating and cruising websites designed for gay men, in which HIV-negative and HIV-positive members navigate around each other as they attempt to find desirable partners. On these websites, prevention of sexually transmitted diseases operates less as a motivating principle for use than a lateral concern that persists in the bodies and apprehensions of members and participants. What is often less apparent in discussions of biological citizenship is the tension between practices of prudence and communal concerns, not to mention the affective repercussions when biological determinations cut through other logics of sociality, sociability, affiliation and belonging. For what is also evident in the accounts given by HIV-negative gay men here are forms of ethical reasoning in which 'care of the self' might initially appear to be at odds with self-protection; in which participants evaluate different practices of HIV prevention in terms of how they might affect others and how they cater to the needs and sensitivities of differently situated participants within shared sexual spaces. Even the younger HIV-negative men interviewed as part of this study can be seen to be engaging in reflexive processes that locate them as participants in a wider sexual culture whose affective dynamics are understood be co-produced and have significant repercussions for others.

At the same time, this chapter reveals some of the mechanisms through which legitimate concerns around self-protection were beginning to materialise into new channels of selective access, partner sorting and socio-sexual exclusion. It is not simply attitudinal prejudice on the part of HIV-negative men, but rather the way in which certain design features were formatting sexual negotiation that began to give rise to what many HIV-positive individuals experienced as a disabling and frustrating affective climate. The concept of affective climates I have begun to elaborate in this chapter helps to conceive how different possibilities of HIV prevention may be understood to emerge as a function of the interactivity of a range of actors – sexual subjects, profile categories, medical information, communicative mechanisms and educational initiatives among them. Indeed, 'care of the self' can be glimpsed here in terms of how it engages the concerns, practices, problems and anticipated performances of a multiplicity of actors, including devices and technologies, so as to contribute to the production of different affective climates. While Foucault's 'technologies of the self' are commonly taken to be individualistic, human-centric processes, this chapter suggests they entail much more than self-interest, and may involve attending to relations among people, devices, categories and things – and problematising them.[4] This underlines the need for better ways of accounting for the activity of non-human actors in what Foucault called 'modes of subjectivation' (Foucault 1990).

The interview material presented in this chapter can be approached for the insight it gives into modes of HIV subjectivation: the processes through which participants make themselves – and are made into – new kinds of subjects of HIV prevention (Foucault 1990; Race 2003). By approaching subjectivation as processual, relational and ongoing, we are better able to conceive the sexual field as dynamic and emergent; to track not simply how sexual subjects incorporate new technologies and discourses into their HIV prevention repertoires, but also how new sexual subjects themselves emerge in relation to ongoing technological developments and convergences (Rosengarten 2010). Such an approach allows us to attend more carefully to the conditions in which new sexual and risk practices materialise, to make out different patterns and possibilities, and to multiply potential sites of constructive intervention. This approach to HIV prevention has certainly been useful in Australia: despite the growing popularity of digital interfaces and the sorting capabilities they afforded, rates of unprotected casual sex among gay men in Sydney defied trends in comparable cities around the world and, rather than increasing, remained relatively stable between 2002 and 2009 – a trend that can arguably be attributed, in part, to educational initiatives addressing the risks and blind-spots of HIV-negative serosorting (Zablotska et al. 2009).

In 2008, Manhunt announced it was upgrading its format. Among the changes was an option to leave the HIV prompt unanswered which had the effect of hiding the HIV status item on members' profiles. The intense discussion surrounding this change among Manhunt members on the company's official blog would seem to indicate some degree of responsiveness to user complaints and suggestions on the part of website developers. As I have discussed in this chapter, online templates shape sexual and risk subjectivities. Little wonder the politics of online formatting and design has emerged as a significant matter of concern for gay men's HIV prevention in the interim.

The updated site also directed members to a separate page called Manhunt Cares through a new Health tab. This page featured links to health resources, information and products available for purchase including diagnostic devices such as HIV home testing kits. These kits (which are available for purchase and delivery in the USA but have not yet been approved for use in Australia) hold the potential to reconfigure gay men's sexual negotiations once again, with a range of effects – both good and bad (Carballo-Diéguez et al. 2012). They may be used to rationalise unprotected sex between HIV-negative individuals, a practice that may give rise to new risks (given the time-lag between infection and the development of HIV antibodies) and pose new sorts of problems and opportunities for sexual partners and sexual community. The possibilities such devices generate by virtue of *what* they make available and *how* indicate the importance of attending to the always local ways in which biomedical, sexual and digital technologies converge and interact to generate material differences in the field of HIV prevention.

Notes

1 At 11pm on a Friday night in November 2008, the Sydney room revealed approximately 920 active users.
2 On the same Friday night in November 2008, the site enumerated 1,150 active users in the Sydney room.

3 This sample – while diverse in terms of age, race, class and other variables – only provides a small qualitative snapshot into what was going on in these cultures and could hardly be considered 'representative' of them in their entirety.
4 On this point I am in agreement with Haraway (2016), who argues that the inextricable entanglement of human and non-human fates that characterises our world requires sympoiesis, (or making-with) rather than autopoiesis (self-making).

References

Ayres, T. 1999. China doll: The experience of being a gay Chinese Australian. *Journal of Homosexuality*, 36(3–4), pp. 87–97.

Callon, M., Y. Millo & Muniesa, F. (eds.) 2007. *Market Devices*. Malden: Blackwell.

Carballo-Diéguez, A., Frasca, T., Balan, I. et al. 2012. Use of a rapid HIV home test prevents HIV exposure in a high-risk sample of men who have sex with men. *AIDS and Behavior*, 16(7), pp. 1753–1760.

Chisolm, D. 2005. *Queer Constellations*. Minneapolis: University of Minnesota Press.

Crimp, D. 1987. How to have promiscuity in an epidemic. *October*, 43, pp. 237–271.

Davis, M., Hart, G., Bolding, G. et al. 2006. E-dating, identity and prevention: theorizing sexualities, risk and network society. *Sociology of Health and Illness*, 28(4), pp. 457–478.

Escoffier, J. 1998. The invention of safer sex: Vernacular knowledge, gay politics and HIV prevention. *Berkeley Journal of Sociology*, 43, pp. 1–30.

Foucault, M., 1990. *The Use of Pleasure: Volume 2 of the History of Sexuality*. Trans. R. Hurley. New York: Vintage Books.

Foucault, M. 1997. Sex, power and the politics of identity. In P. Rabinow (ed.) *Ethics: Subjectivity and Truth*. London: Penguin, pp. 163–174.

Halperin, D. 2007. *What Do Gay Men Want? An Essay on Sex, Risk, and Subjectivity*. Ann Arbor: University of Michigan Press.

Han, A. 2006. 'I think you're the smartest race I've ever met': Racialised economies of queer male desire. *Australian Critical Race & Whiteness Studies Association ejournal*, 2(2), pp. 1–14.

Haraway, D. 2016. *Staying with the Trouble: Making Kin in the Chthulucene*. Durham: Duke University Press.

Hardey, M. 2002. Life beyond the screen: Embodiment and identity through the Internet. *The Sociological Review*, 50(4), pp. 571–585.

Hoppe, T. 2017. *Punishing Disease*. Berkley: University of California Press.

Kippax, S., Crawford, J., Davis, M., et al. 1993. Sustaining safe sex: A longitudinal study of a sample of homosexual men. *AIDS*, 7(2), pp. 257–264.

Kippax, S. & Race, K. 2003. Sustaining safe practice: Twenty years on. *Social Science & Medicine*, 57(1), pp. 1–12.

Latour, B. 2004. How to talk about the body? The normative dimension of science studies. *Body & Society*, 10(2–3), pp. 205–229.

Mansfield, T. & Quan, A. 2006. *Sexual racism sux* [online]. Retrieved from https://sexualracismsux.com [27 January 2017].

Ong, A. & Collier, S. (eds.) 2005. *Global Assemblages: Technology, Politics, and Ethics as Anthropological Problems*. Oxford: Blackwell.

Patton, C. 1990. *Inventing AIDS*. New York: Routledge.

Race, K., 2001. The undetectable crisis: Changing technologies of risk. *Sexualities*, 4(2), pp. 167–189.

Race, K. 2003. Revaluation of risk among gay men. *AIDS Education & Prevention*, 15(4), pp. 369–381.

Rose, N. & Novas, C. 2005. Biological citizenship. In A. Ong & S. Collier (eds.) *Global Assemblages: Technology, Politics, and Ethics as Anthropological Problems*. Oxford: Blackwell, pp. 440–463.

Rosengarten, M., 2010. *HIV Interventions: Biomedicine and the Traffic between Information and Flesh*. Seattle, WA: University of Washington Press.

Sendziuk, P. 2003. *Learning to Trust: Australian Responses to HIV/AIDS*. Sydney: UNSW Press.

Van Zoonen, L. 2002. Gendering the Internet: Claims, Controversies and Cultures. *European Journal of Communication*, 17(1), pp. 5–23.

Warner, M. 2000. *The Trouble with Normal*. Cambridge, MA: Harvard University Press.

Watney, S. 1988. *Policing Desire*. Minneapolis: University of Minnesota Press.

Zablotska, I., Prestage, G., Frankland, A. et al. 2007. *Sydney Gay Community Periodic Survey, February 1996–August 2006*. Sydney: National Centre in HIV Social Research.

Zablotska, I., Prestage, G., Frankland, A., et al. 2008. *Gay Community Periodic Survey*. Sydney: National Centre in HIV Social Research.

Zablotska, I., Imrie, J., Prestage, G. et al. 2009. Gay men's current practice of HIV seroconcordant unprotected anal intercourse: Serosorting or seroguessing?. *AIDS Care*, 21(4), pp. 501–510.

4   Making up barebackers

In his book *Autopornography*, the HIV-positive gay pornstar, writer and sex advocate Scott O'Hara provides a frank and amiable account of his sexual experience during the first phase of the AIDS epidemic in North America (O'Hara 1997a). He describes periods of abstinence, of limiting his sexual practice to certain acts (both alone and with particular partners), of using condoms for anal sex (on one occasion he describes this as 'kinky' and 'hot') and also of unprotected sex. He describes times when he had no libido at all, some of which coincide with periods of illness, and he describes a time after 1994 when his libido returns, when he realises 'there were other HIVers out there with whom I didn't need to worry about transmission; men who didn't worry about isolating bodily fluids' (1997a, p. 129). Despite his upfront sexual manner and sexual articulacy, O'Hara relates how he found it difficult to raise the subject of AIDS with potential sex partners, such that he'd 'essentially given up sex rather than learn[ed] to discuss it' (1997a, p. 127). In 1994, he gets an 'HIV+' tattoo on his left bicep (which he refers to as the most visible spot on his body save his forehead) and surrounds it with a 'tasteful little circlet of swimming spermatozoa'. These steps are taken in an attempt to ensure that the sex he has is safe or at least better informed with respect to HIV transmission. For example, on one occasion he describes a sexual encounter with a 'redneck' where he avoids doing anything risky (even oral sex) because it is too dark to see his tattoo. He suggests they jerk each other off in a scene he describes as 'really exciting' (1997a, p. 200).

Although not all gay men are pornstars or poets, O'Hara's thinking here is typical of the concerns and innovations expressed by many HIV-positive gay men (Adam 2005; Rosengarten et al. 2000). He takes care not to put HIV-negative men at risk, and because of his preference for sex without condoms he tries to ensure his sexual partners are other HIV-positive men. He describes the risk of sexually transmitted infections and 'possibly other things that are transmissible among HIVers too', but places little emphasis on these possibilities. 'I assume my partner has the same deductive facilities that I have so I grant him the right to make his own decisions about what precautions he thinks are appropriate' (1997a, p. 201). O'Hara is also alert to the way in which risk and health discourses can be used to naturalise and promote certain moral regimes. At one point, he voices his suspicion that the medical profession's fixation on these dangers 'has more to do with its longstanding distaste for gay sex than on scientific research. You know: Anal Sex – Icky! Dirty!'. Believing some doctors to be 'only too happy to make whatever judgments they can to stop people from having dirty, messy sex', he suggests 'people just need to learn what their own personal safety guidelines are. I doubt the medical profession will offer much realistic help along those lines, so it's up to us to use our noggins' (1997a, p. 202).

Elsewhere, however, these risks play a more constitutive role in O'Hara's erotic negotiations with other HIV-positive men:

> Nowadays when I make an agreement with a man that we'll fuck uncovered, it's an extreme declaration of trust, knowing that there are potentially lethal diseases that we could be passing back and forth – crypto, meningitis, hepatitis – and we think it's worth the risk.

Though he reports only four instances of this sort of occasion, 'each time stands out, diamond sharp, in my memory, more because of the trust shared than because the sex was extra special' (1997a, p. 202). Without necessarily objecting to these instances, it is worth observing that if the stakes of intimacy can be raised in this way, it would seem the risks have made some impression.

O'Hara's account offers a valuable record of some of the ways gay men have negotiated different and sometimes contradictory formations of sex, infection, risk, responsibility and intimacy. He provides a candid and unapologetic account of the variable positions in which he finds himself as a gendered subject of medical, sexual and romantic discourses. Perhaps what is most confronting in O'Hara's writings for those concerned with HIV prevention is his refusal to subordinate his self-esteem to the prerogatives of HIV prevention. While he never endorses recklessness on the part of HIV-positive individuals, he is not prepared to let public health imperatives determine his self-conception as a gay man with a particular relation to HIV:

> I've become somewhat notorious, over the past year, for my positions on HIV. To put it briefly as possible: I can't quite believe it's a curse. I'm not trying to out-Louise Ms. Hay, but in my life, AIDS has been an undeniable blessing. It woke me up to what was important; it let me know that NOW was the time to do it. And – this is the part that upsets people – it also gives me the freedom to behave 'irresponsibly'. I look at the HIV negative people around me, and I pity them. They live their lives in constant fear of infection: mustn't do this, mustn't do that, mustn't take risks. They can't see past that simple 'avoidance of infection', which has come to be their ultimate goal. They believe that AIDS=death sentence. Well, I'm sorry, but I was quite possibly infected in 1981, and I'm in pretty good health 15 years later. If that's a death sentence, I guess life

in a prison of negativity sounds a lot worse. My life is so much more carefree than theirs, so much more 'considered', that I shake my head and count myself lucky to have been infected. Risk taking is the essence of life, and people who spend their entire lives trying to eliminate risk from their lives are . . . well, they're not my kind of people. I know a couple of people who have self-consciously made the decision to seroconvert; I admire them tremendously, because it takes a considerable amount of self-confidence and self-knowledge to make a decision that flies in the face of every medical and journalistic opinion in the world. I applaud this sort of independence. These men are, I might add, some of the most inventive sex partners I've been with. No surprise.

(1997a, p. 129)

The final sentences of this passage enable us to imagine how becoming infected might emerge for some people as a considered solution (though not an ideal or common one) to a problem experienced by them as insufferable: having to live a life hounded by persistent anxieties about HIV infection.

It is illustrative of O'Hara's position as a minoritised sexual and medical subject that his sexual practice entails practices of cultural production. To create a viable context for his life, he found himself contending with forces that would keep both homosexuality and the realities of HIV isolated and private. Although he spent most of his career writing about, discussing and practising sex, at the heart of O'Hara's work as a cultural producer is a conviction that there is nothing very special about it. In the preface to *Autopornography* he writes, 'sex is really not the all important subject that my writing would seem to imply', though he admits to having had a 'one-string harp for the past decade'.

All I want is for sex and porn to take their proper places in life, alongside eating and writing letters – enjoyable activities, not for everyone perhaps, but normal, beneficial, and quite, quite harmless to children. Nothing to get excited about.

(1997a, p. ix)

For O'Hara, sex is a field of friendly sociability and ordinary belonging. Indeed, when he wants to convey his attitude to sex in his later videos, he does something quite unusual in gay porn: he smiles. In 1993, O'Hara established *Steam* magazine, a publication he edited and billed as a 'Quarterly Journal for Men'. The magazine featured accounts of his and other writers' sexual experiences, as well as reports on bathhouses and other areas where gay men meet for sex, alongside various commentary and writing on sexual matters. Among the contents were regular discussions of HIV issues, though these were not restricted to unexamined rehearsals of public health mantra. *Steam* contributed to what had become a flourishing public culture around sexuality in the USA and elsewhere, only one of a multitude of circulars, events, meeting places, conferences, performances, parties and collections that offered alternatives to the authorised construction of sex as rightfully situated in the home, between man and wife, in the context of conjugal intimacy. Like other projects of this sort, the magazine hoped to reverse the damaging disinformation of privacy and shame that produces and suffocates subordinated sexualities. Thus, whatever problems one might have with the way in which O'Hara positions HIV seroconversion in the passage above (where the decision is praised for its bravado, independence and exemplification of masculine sexual prowess), one can also appreciate the way he helped activate a public setting in which such issues could be debated and collectively negotiated.

I have opened this chapter with a discussion of Scott O'Hara's work as a way into some of the historic dimensions of HIV-related subjectivation among gay and other men who have sex with men. O'Hara's discourse is reminiscent of a certain approach to sex one often encountered in urban gay cultures in various parts of the world in the wake of gay liberation and queer politics. I do not wish to overstate or lionise O'Hara's celebrity, since to do so would be to frame him in terms of some norm or ideality when what I seek is a more ethical engagement with the corpus of material from which his work is drawn. Indeed I find myself in the curious position of wanting at once to affirm and resist O'Hara's authority. O'Hara was only one of several voices that began to speak and write of the pleasures of unprotected sex at about the time that combination antiretroviral therapy was made available in the West (1997b). These accounts typically referred to unprotected penetrative sex between HIV-positive men – something that is safe with respect to HIV transmission.[1] But because they breached established norms around safe sex and the use of condoms, these declarations were subject to considerable alarm and moral panic in some locations and attacked as irresponsible by many critics.

I want to affirm such accounts in that they represent creative and situated experiments with possible configurations of HIV prevention and sexual pleasure. They contribute to a larger project of collective self-improvisation that has been crucial to the success of HIV prevention and from which the original invention of 'safe sex' sprang. By attending to the situated experience of sex and risk, accounts such as O'Hara's mobilise lay knowledge for the construction of viable intimate practices that aim to avoid HIV transmission. Rather than positioning risk and safety as fixed practices, they tackle the more difficult work of conceiving of HIV risk as subject to relational dynamics that typically involve intimate negotiation between two or more persons as well as changing technologies and conditions. They approach risk as a matter of creative responsiveness and interpersonal sensemaking rather than regulatory prescription by technocrats. The authority to define risk and safety is wrestled away from medical monopoly and opened up onto a public and popularly accessible sphere. I believe such an approach is potentially of great value to those who wish to promote some movement around HIV prevention.

Another reason for citing O'Hara here is that he is often associated with – and sometimes even attributed authorship of – a specific valuation of unprotected anal sex known as barebacking. Indeed, he comes close to claiming this authority for himself when he says in a 1997 opinion piece that he was 'probably the first person to make a public Declaration of Intent to Engage in Unsafe Sex in a national publication' (O'Hara 1997b).[2] Barebacking emerged in the context of a series of accounts of this sort that provoked outrage both within and outside the gay press, such that it soon took on the sense of an 'erotically charged, premeditated act' with little reference to the question of HIV serostatus, and in some instances a highly sensationalised investment in 'risk' (Rofes 1998).[3] I am interested in the conditions in which self-accounts such as O'Hara's can be taken to amount to a defiant and indiscriminate intentionality with respect to HIV transmission, as well as the sense in which those conditions can be understood as disciplinary.[4] I want to suggest that barebacking can be approached as the outcome of a fractious encounter between normative morality and embodied ethics in which the latter were basically misrecognised by the former. O'Hara's is a pedagogical instance because of the ethical care (and also self-regard) that can be found in his sexual practice. By tracking the different forms his discourse takes as it moves from one scene of publicity to another, we can see how barebacking takes on a life of its own and how this investment in 'unsafe sex' depends on an encounter between normative apprehension and a defensive response to this apprehension, such that the desire for sex without condoms materialises occasionally as a defiant intent to have *unsafe* sex. In making what could be regarded as a perfectly viable proposal around HIV-positive sexual practice, barebacking reached for what is perhaps the most available language to defend a practice under attack: the language of individual rights and entitlements. This had the effect of framing sex without condoms as a property or entitlement rather than a relation between people, promoting what some have analysed as a presumptive disregard of the other within barebacking discourse (Adam 2005). It is O'Hara's defensive, individualised citation of the norm and the way it encourages us to relate to sex as an abstract property or entitlement rather than a relational field that I wish to resist. Thus I propose to use O'Hara's writings and their circulation as an entry point into a broader analysis of the normative conditions in which HIV-positive sexual practice becomes uncovered.

'An intimacy previously missing'

Some insight into these conditions can be gleaned from an article that appeared in the *San Francisco Chronicle* in February 2006 entitled 'The Same Sex Scene: A Serosorting Story' (Heredia 2006). Despite the inflammatory reaction to barebacking in 1997, an apparent decline in the rate of new infections in San Francisco by 2006 despite increases in so-called 'risk practice' led some authorities to embrace what they called 'serosorting' – the practice of selecting sexual partners on the basis of sharing the same HIV status.

This is of course the same practice that people like O'Hara were promoting in the furore over barebacking, although now respectabilised some ten years later with a scientific designation (the irony of which is underscored in the comments of one man interviewed for this article: 'I was doing serosorting before they had a word for it. Now, they're saying it is an effective prevention strategy, which is great'). But where barebacking became a scandal by virtue of its apparent association with promiscuity and casual sex, serosorting is normalised within this article with reference to a conjugal frame that promises 'an intimacy previously missing'.[5] By paying attention to the terms in which serosorting is endorsed for a mainstream audience, we can gain insight into some of the forces that mediate the intelligibility of gay sex as it bears on HIV prevention. What is interesting is that while barebacking and serosorting clearly overlap (and may actually refer to the same thing in practice), they proclaim quite different positions in the field of sexual morality, revealing how risk discourse gets filtered through more traditional moral categories. Where barebacking foregrounds desire and sensation and is not always explicit about the concern for HIV prevention that often informs the practice, this article frames serosorting in terms of HIV prevention and risk avoidance, but ends up promoting an oddly desexualised image.

Serosorting is constructed in the article as a form of mutual support ('leaning on each other') in the context of chronic illness, with the added spin-off of HIV containment. The story opens with a 'waiting room romance' at the clinic where two long-term HIV survivors meet and fall in love. The article situates serosorting in terms of some of the pressures that bear on HIV-positive subjectivity, with the HIV-positive individuals interviewed speaking of the stresses associated with the fear of infecting others, the challenges of disclosing HIV status to new partners and the advantages of negotiating elements of long-term chronic illness in relation with someone who knows what to expect and who is going through something similar. For these individuals, seroconcordant relations are one way of resolving such concerns. The article cites a San Francisco couples' therapist, who suggests that HIV-positive men are not hooking up to help the community so much as avoiding having to disclose their status to (potentially unsympathetic) partners, and to have sex without condoms. The physiological changes associated with the use of early protease inhibitors, and the whole process of having to hide or explain one's medications, are things that many HIV-positive individuals would prefer to avoid, he explains. 'In serosorting they're looking for somebody who doesn't have issues with these things'. These comments anchor serosorting within practices of HIV-positive subjectification, casting it as a reasonable response to historic configurations of risk, responsibility, pleasure, health and pharmaceutical regimes. But when serosorting is seized upon as an acceptable HIV prevention strategy, something funny happens. The story quotes interview material from Lee, a forty-four-year-old part-time usher who 'prefers to only date HIV-positive men because he would rather have sex without condoms'. The emergence of HIV dating sites on the Internet and the high proportion of

HIV-positive gay men in San Francisco are cited as conditions that enable him to disclose his HIV status easily. The inclusion of Lee is noteworthy because his sex life does not adhere strictly to the ideal of long-term conjugal commitment. But Lee is drawn in the heterosexual imagery of 'dating' ('I exclusively date HIV-positive guys'), and is pictured spending time with his partners engaging in couple-like activities such as going to the movies.

Meanwhile, James and Brian, the feature couple of the article, are monogamous. The article probes their intimate life, claiming the couple's sex life has 'evolved'. Though at first they had sex without condoms, concerns about superinfection prompted changes in their sexual practice. They now 'enjoy kissing, petting, preening and massaging each other . . . "To be in love with somebody and having a fulfilling life you're not missing out on anything not having penetrative sex"', one of the pair is quoted as saying. The article closes with the couple gently caressing and snuggling on the couch, highlighting their 'matching titanium rings'. 'The only time we're apart is when we're on our way to getting together'.

The construction of serosorting in this article brings home the significance of attending to the ways in which practices involving gay sex and HIV prevention are normatively understood. Where barebacking was misrecognised as intentional recklessness such that the practical ethics informing the practice were lost in translation, serosorting is celebrated in conventional terms that invisibilise gay practices and cultures of casual sex. It is telling that the valorisation of serosorting in this piece rests on the ultimate erasure of gay anal sex as well as an invocation of matrimonial ideals. A normative investment in segregation also becomes apparent in some of the discourse the article cites: 'Seroselecting is like choosing somebody who is in the same church, like being Episcopalian or Methodist and wanting to marry an Episcopalian or Methodist . . . . They just get it, you don't have to explain'. There are times in this article when serosorting appears to be nothing more than an intricate device through which gay men might be shepherded into normative modes of relationship, sorted by HIV status. The narrative exudes a certain phobia around the very idea of sexually active HIV-positive people (see Crimp 1992). But this characteristic only indicates a more immediate problem for HIV prevention workers who must come up with realistic strategies adapted to the practical contexts in which gay sex occurs.

While the discourse of serosorting references a widely accessible (and widely accessed) culture of casual sex, it offers a somewhat sanitised version that does not exactly correspond with the sexual culture in which most serosorting takes place. In all the talk around serosorting, there is little attention to the relational or situational contexts of gay sex or their practical contingencies. While the apparent anonymity of the Internet may have made it easier for some HIV-positive men to disclose their status when seeking sex online, disclosure remained rare in many of the contexts in which gay sex occurred at this time, and there are considerable obstacles and practical difficulties around disclosure for HIV-positive gay men (Sheon & Crosby 2004). Meanwhile, in social research a surprising number of HIV-negative men indicate rarely knowingly having sex with an HIV-positive partner (a claim not likely to reflect reality) and it seems few HIV-negative men are clued into the sometimes very subtle attempts of HIV-positive men to negotiate seroconcordant unprotected sex, many of which do not involve spoken disclosure of HIV status (Van de Ven et al. 2001; Adam 2005). In this sense, the discourse of serosorting may promote a certain brand of wishful thinking that is much more difficult to enact in practice. While finding ways in which gay men can safely enjoy unprotected anal sex (including in casual contexts) is important, the uncovering of gay sex within this discourse is premised upon a normative misrecognition of much gay sexual practice and promotes similar misrecognition *within* it, raising its own set of challenges and risks.

The appearance of the Internet in this narrative dramatises some of the paradoxes of normative exposure for HIV-positive subjects and brings us back to the discussion of O'Hara. For while norms of individual responsibility would seem to require that HIV-positive subjects advertise their status when seeking sex online, it is just such an advertisement that some HIV prevention advocates fretted about, with the Internet positioned as a 'reason' for unsafe sex in some accounts (Halkitis & Parsons 2003). In the context of barebacking, the Internet was often said to cause risk by virtue of the visibility it gave to HIV-positive sex, but in the context of serosorting it becomes an icon of responsibility. The terms of risk become identifiable with the terms of responsibility here, insofar as both anticipate some level of self-publicity around HIV-positive status. It is noteworthy, for example, that O'Hara cites national publicity as the context for his Declaration of Intent. The norms of abstract personhood that inhere in the national public sphere led him to discount the relational or embodied contexts of his practice (HIV-positive seroconcordance) in favour of an assertion of his individual entitlement.[6] O'Hara's self-disclosure can similarly be understood to involve a certain 'taking' of responsibility. His sexual practice is taken in normative terms to be 'irresponsible', though a more detailed account reveals that it is carefully considered. Normative constructions of responsibility work to undercut ethical relations to the self and others here and spectacularise them as risk. At this moment, we can see how risk and responsibility enter into a zone of indistinction for HIV subjects and it becomes apparent that barebacking and serosorting run the same range of risks, alternatively grasped: the normative misrecognition of provisional practices of responsibility. Perhaps what needs to be contended with here is the sensationalising discourse of the public sphere that turns minor instances of self-disclosure into advertisements.[7]

By considering these media in terms of how they work to construct various public and counterpublic identities and subjectivities, we gain insight into how different risks materialise around HIV and what this has to do with mass publicity. If we consider that bodies only make sense within a disciplinary frame shot through with sex and gender norms, we can ask how a sexed and gendered 'grid of intelligibility' mediates the ways in which various responses to HIV become available,[8] and the difference that different scenes of publicity make to their materialisation. What happens as various parties strive to make minoritised practices (of HIV risk but also HIV prevention) normatively intelligible? What distortions, impasses, identities, advantages and compromises ensue and how are these negotiated? The combination of minoritised sexuality, mass abstraction and discipline at play here suggests the need to theorise ways in which experience can be grasped as particular, and particularly shared. I am interested therefore in the question of how to engage with barebacking, and how one might engage critically with this body of material without inciting the same defiant charge. My hope is to perform a different relation to the body of material from which O'Hara's voices are drawn – one that is not confined to the binary terms of moral denunciation and liberal celebration.

The disciplinary production of 'intentional' unsafe sex

I stated above that this analysis concerns the disciplinary conditions in which gay sex involving HIV-positive subjects becomes uncovered. I meant to suggest the ways in which normative constraints on the representation of gay sex and HIV might be considered implicated in the proliferation of barebacking. It bears emphasising, however, that barebacking is only one of the descriptions gay men give for unprotected sex, and individual 'intention' only one of the explanations. In Australia, for example, education has been conducted on how to ensure safe unprotected sex between HIV-negative gay men in regular relationships since 1994 (dubbed 'negotiated safety') in a move that may arguably have undermined some of the appeal of so-called 'barebacking' (see Chapter 1, and Kippax 2002). Apart from this and similar risk reduction practices, gay men account for unsafe sex in a number of ways (Adam 2005): erectile difficulty or frustration with condoms, getting carried away with the moment, slipping up, mistaken assumptions about their partner's HIV status, desiring greater intimacy or intensity, particular relational dynamics (such as not wanting to compromise the encounter because of the partner's presumed superiority and/or desire for unprotected sex), not knowing how to introduce a condom, being drunk or out of it on drugs, forgetting, an accident, personal turmoil – and this is only the beginning of an interminable list, none of which are necessarily best understood as either 'barebacking' or 'intentional'.

Wanting greater precision in their documentation of the offending practice, social scientists soon came to define barebacking more strictly as 'intentional unsafe sex' (Halkitis & Parsons 2003). But as Gregory Tomso observed, this move to define barebacking as 'intentional unsafe sex' had the effect of producing barebacking as a problem of volition and desire, generating even greater policing and scrutiny of gay men's moral intentions (Tomso 2004). Meanwhile, even among self-identified barebackers the most common explanation given for their 'intentions' was wanting greater physical stimulation and wanting to feel emotionally connected to their partner.

Only 17 per cent of a sample of HIV-negative 'barebackers' from San Francisco gave as their reason wanting to 'do something taboo or racy', while 22 per cent cited their motivation 'to take a major risk' (these items were not mutually exclusive) (Mansergh et al. 2002).[9]

Admittedly, surveys are a blunt instrument when it comes to investigating the complexity of subjective meanings, but it would seem that on this definition the eroticisation of risk counts for only a small portion of self-reported barebacking. The subject of my analysis though is not the actual prevalence of eroticised risk in the gay population (which appears to be limited), but *the processes through which unsafe sex materialises as a matter of defiant intention*. I understand eroticised risk as the mainly unrealised potential of concrete processes of subjectivation. These processes could be understood as disciplinary in that they involve the recognition of some level of agency and desire in the vicinity of risk (e.g. a desire for sex without condoms), a normative confrontation or condemnation of that agency and an aggravated response to that confrontation. My focus, in other words, is on the refraction of individual desire through official discourses that responsibilise the subject.[10] I query the system that would erotically construct gay men as intentional deviants when it comes to HIV transmission. As Tomso observes, one cannot separate out 'media representations' and 'scientific facts' here; the conflation of barebacking with other instances of unprotected sex takes place in both the media and scientific discourse (Tomso 2004). And since HIV is such a dense site of positivist social science, I turn now to a consideration of some of the ways in which social science participates in this risky process of responsibilisation.

A 2003 study sets out to assess 'the frequency with which gay and bisexual men in New York City engage in intentional unprotected sex, or "barebacking"' (Halkitis et al. 2003). The authors set up their report with some precision. They begin by noting that unprotected anal sex has 'gained momentum' in the last several years 'in part because of relapse from safer sex on the part of gay and bisexual men, but also to [sic] the increasingly popular behavioural phenomenon of intentional unsafe sex, referred to as "barebacking"' (2003, p. 351). They acknowledge that 'intentional unsafe anal acts may yield minimal or no risk' of HIV transmission in the context of seroconcordant partnerships: unprotected sex between two people known to be of the same HIV status poses no risk of HIV infection. And they discuss the need (by now registered in the science) to differentiate between 'unintentional' unsafe behaviour and 'the increasingly popular unsafe anal practices, which are "intentional" and/ or premeditated', and are said to be 'colloquially known in the mainstream and academic press as "barebacking"' (2003, p. 352). This initial meticulousness bears an ambiguous relation to the study's method, however, which the authors outline as follows:

> Participants were asked to respond to the following questions: I am familiar with the term 'barebacking' as it is used by gay men to describe their sexual behavior. No further definition of the 'barebacking' was provided

to participants by the research team as we were interested in individual perceptions of the phenomenon; however, 'barebacking' was clearly identified by the survey as a term related to the sexual practices of gay men. Our previous work has shown that barebacking is typically understood by gay men in NYC to refer to intentional unprotected anal intercourse. If they reported familiarity with the term, participants were then asked to report the number of men with whom they had engaged in bareback sex in the 3 months prior to assessment.

(2003, p. 353)

This method yielded the finding that 45.5 per cent of the 448 men familiar with the term barebacking reported engaging in bareback sex with at least one sexual partner in the previous three months[11] – a figure that is considerably higher than the 14 per cent reported in a 2002 San Francisco study that defined barebacking more strictly as 'intentional unprotected anal intercourse with a non-primary partner' (Mansergh et al. 2002). On the basis of these findings and reported increases in HIV seroconversion, the authors claim that 'intentional unprotected sex is increasing among gay and bisexual men' (Halkitis et al. 2003).

To be fair, the meaning of the term 'barebacking' depends on its usage and circulation. It is not set in time, fixed once and for all. Indeed, the method of this study could be considered well attuned to the dynamics of the floating signifier: it is necessary and perhaps important for researchers to investigate everyday perceptions and usages of cultural terms which may be much wider and more various after all than any 'original' definition. In other words, it is quite probable that the term 'barebacking' had travelled well beyond any initial definition by this time and was being used loosely by many gay men to refer to sex without condoms in general. (This might explain the fact that half the sample reported engaging in barebacking – a figure that resembles rates of unprotected sex in this location at this time.) That said, there is a tension here between what the study claims to be doing and what it actually does. In particular, it secretly narrows the definition of the term 'barebacking' even as it casts a wide net around the meaning of the term for study participants. Through its prefatory definitional work, the study captured as 'intentional unprotected sex' what might in fact be a considerably more diverse range of practices and occasions. It misrecognises the vernacular of participants as completely identifiable with the term as it was scientifically defined, and encourages the subject of this discourse to misrecognise it too. In this sense, the study does indeed offer a convincing 'Explanation for the Emergence of Intentional Unsafe Behavior', as it claims to in the subtitle: the constitutive and normalising work of HIV social science itself! The steps it takes are intimately involved in the misrecognition and materialisation of gay sex without condoms as a matter of *intention*.

In making this claim, my aim is not to write off HIV social research in general, or these researchers in particular, who certainly make a productive contribution to understandings of HIV risk. Rather, my concern is that this mode of enquiry actually promotes a subtle misrecognition of the contingencies of practice, such that gay men are encouraged to recognise as a matter of 'intention' something that may in fact be much more variable. This is not to argue that gay men are not accountable for what happens in the various sexual contexts in which they find themselves; rather, the point is that this mode of identification encourages a turning away from the contingencies of sexual and risk relations, when what could otherwise be promoted is more careful consideration of them. My claim is that this mode of accountability, this crafting of an intentional individual subject of risk – which is as much a corollary of social scientific practice as it is of wider discourse – does not adequately address the circumstances and the matter at hand.

To explore this point further, let us turn to a valuable discussion of the talk of recently diagnosed HIV-positive gay men in Sydney. In a perceptive analysis, Sean Slavin and colleagues (2004) discuss the range of accounts of unprotected sex that participants believed to have put them at risk. These include an account of attempted risk reduction among serodiscordant partners; an account involving sex with an attractive partner while on the recreational drug ecstasy; an account of 'not caring what happened' and intense feelings of passion and intimacy; and an account involving wanting to 'make things easy' in the context of a relationship with an HIV-positive partner. As the authors discuss, '[t]hese four men narrate their experience of risk not as a result of an accident or misinformation, but as individual choices, informed about risk. Informed, that is, about the technical principles and "objective" facts of viral transmission':

> They all claim to have known what they were doing at the time of infection and had made a choice, freely and rationally. They all attempt to distinguish between these principles of choice and any emotional, social and cultural context in which they are situated . . . . There is a sense in all these narratives that participants hold themselves solely responsible for having become infected, that they knew what they were doing. They do not consider that context or other factors beyond their control may have mediated the decisions they were making. Such an acknowledgement would seem to question their belief in themselves as 'in control' – of themselves and their circumstances.
>
> (2004, p. 45)

The authors treat these characteristics as a feature of the discourse or experience of this 'group' of individuals, but what if we were to approach these features as an effect of the disciplinary grid through which these subjects are led to recognise themselves as subjects? Each of these accounts is made in the context of an open-ended interview conducted a short time after seroconversion. Participants were referred to the study by their HIV clinician and interviewed by a social researcher, either at home or at a community health centre. It is difficult to say whether the context of a private interview gives the participant more or less opportunity to explore their experience in tentative terms – most likely it differs from case to case. But it is interesting to consider what sort of subject is produced in this specific relational context. As the authors discuss, this is a subject who is rational and decisional and in control of their circumstances, whose choice with respect to risk exists outside any relational or temporal setting (2004, p. 48). Thus, while participants give fairly fluent accounts of the circumstances they believe placed them at risk, they also insist, as the authors report, on a rational, choice-making self. In particular, they discount the effects of these circumstances on what they call their 'decisions about risk'. These accounts can be read as records of a process of subjectivation constrained by certain norms of intelligibility: they give clues to the sort of subject that emerges as a product of authoritative discourse. Are these individuals participants in acts of 'intentional unsafe sex'? Only within a disciplinary frame that invites them to recognise themselves as such. While it would be possible to argue for the need for a subject even *more* in control of their circumstances given the possibility of HIV infection in these instances, it is worth considering that such an approach might actually promote further occlusion of the complex relations that make up sexual events and sexual lives.

In his study of the discourses of HIV-positive men in Toronto who use the language of barebacking to describe their practice, Barry Adam finds that

> interviews with self-professed barebackers reveal not so much rebellion or transgression as something more prosaic and more consistent with the discourses of government and capital. Not only does the responsibilisation message resonate throughout their own accounts but the larger rhetoric of neoliberalism does as well, of which responsibility talk is a part.
>
> (Adam 2005)

Adam's analysis deals only with HIV-positive barebackers, who might be expected to bear a different relation to the erotics of risk than those *at risk* of HIV infection. He situates barebacking as a personal policy found among some HIV-positive men within urban gay communities embedded in a larger context of encountering men who are HIV-positive or 'in the know'. As is evident in O'Hara's accounts of his sexual practice, neither the practical morality nor the actual practices of the HIV-positive men interviewed 'overtly intend HIV transmission to happen' (2005, p. 341).[12] But as Adam illustrates, their practice relies on extremely subtle negotiations that HIV-negative men are often unaware of and which may not allow for the complex 'vulnerabilities, emotions and tough dilemmas' that characterise sexual interaction (2005, p. 344).

One of the values of Adam's study is the way it illustrates how the discourse of barebackers is consonant with wider, dominant discourses that structure social life and moral reasoning. 'In many ways', Adam writes, these accounts of unsafe sex participate in the moral reasoning widely propagated by government and business today that constructs each as a self-interested individual who must take responsibility for himself in a marketplace of risks. It is perhaps also a particularly masculine discourse in its evocation of norms of competitive individualism.

(2005, p. 340)

However, unlike so many accounts of gay life circulating even in leftist circles today, Adam does not hold gay men up as exemplars of neoliberal ideology. Rather, he remains alive to the virtualities of subject formation, suggesting, for example, that 'neoliberal discourse is not totalising nor does it capture the subjectivity of these men in a fundamental way', and pointing to competing discourses 'drawn from romance, masculine adventure, gay solidarity, communitarianism, and so on, that can come to the fore, according to circumstance' (2005, p. 345). By appealing to gay men to take care of other men '(instead of simply defending themselves against other men)', he locates his critique within a tradition of gendered counter-practice:

It would be an appeal that would run against leading ideologies in circulation in our society today but one that would likely have considerable resonance among men whose sexual pursuits are often linked with the desire to love and be loved by other men.

(2005, p. 345)

Especially useful in this regard is the way Adam's methodology undercuts some of the epistemological and ideological commitments of neoliberalism. He recognises and documents the moral intentions of his subjects but also finds ways of suggesting that a mere focus on *intentions* is not the end of a practical response. In this sense, his analysis moves in precisely the opposite direction to the discourses discussed above, which totalise the question of intention while ignoring the circumstances of prevention. Rather than debunking neoliberal ideologies in a familiar critical style, Adam recognises their sedimentation in the embodied experience of study participants and gestures towards other tendencies and possibilities. The ethical sensibilities of participants can thus become involved in a wider querying of normative frameworks of personhood. With its emphasis on the constitutive work of wider moral ideologies, this study offers a better basis for an ethical engagement with barebacking, insofar as it gestures towards more open possibilities of subject formation.

Barebacking: real time

Throughout this chapter I have been concerned with the disciplinary technologies through which gay men are made into subjects of HIV prevention. I have argued that in making themselves and being made into such, gay men have been led to interpret certain of their sexual activities and desires as intentional deviance with respect to HIV risk, and this leads to a misrecognition of the preventive possibilities of their practice. This process can be understood as an effect, in part, of the disciplinary grid through which HIV subjectivities were produced in the first decade of the millennium. My suggestion is that more flexible modes of attention to the circumstances of sex, pleasure and HIV prevention may offset the materialisation of barebacking as an intentional act reducible to the eroticisation of HIV transmission.

This is not to deny the circulation of eroticised expressions of HIV transmission in gay male pornography and online discourse at this time. The sexual imagination is highly versatile and endlessly inventive, and it should come as no surprise that one response to the fear of HIV transmission has been to eroticise it. Numerous studies from the early 2000s point to a fascination with the discourses of 'bug-chasing' and 'gift-giving' in their analyses of online profile ads and gay pornography (Grov 2004; Tewksbury 2006; Dean 2008, 2009). These studies typically approach barebacking as an exotic or foreign subculture with its own set of meanings that can be gleaned from virtual expressions of barebacking fantasies. As informative and imaginative as these studies often are, in general they show little interest in the social pragmatics of sex and pleasure. Even the most brilliant tend to downplay the significance of certain distinctions that are highly material to many participants in barebacking subculture – between unprotected sex and HIV transmission; between serodiscordant and seroconcordant sex; between fantasy and practice. Indeed, more often than not, these studies are caught up in what Foucault called the *hermeneutics of desire*; 'Tell me what your desire is, and I'll tell you who you are' (Foucault 2011, p. 389). They totalise and individualise barebacking as an anti-normative identity by reducing it entirely to obscure expressions of desire. But as I have argued, the signification of barebacking is much looser and less unified than these studies tend to find. Indeed, barebacking is a much more heterogenous domain of problematisation, insofar as it embodies a complex ensemble of difficulties 'to which diverse solutions are proposed' (Ong & Collier 2005, p. 43). Deliberate HIV infection is only one potential solution to the ensemble of difficulties that barebacking attempts to address – a point whose significance becomes obvious when considering one of the flagship instantiations of barebacking culture worldwide.

Founded in 2004, the online cruising site BareBackRealTime.com (BBRT) describes itself as 'the world's largest hookup site for men looking for other barebackers' (Pigmaster 2008). In an interview with its founder, it emerges that BBRT was established in response to the sort of HIV-positive disaffection with mainstream cruising sites discussed in Chapter 3. As Pigmaster (the pseudonymous founder of BBRT) explains in this interview,

> I started the site out of frustration that when dealing with other websites when you filled in your status as HIV, people were freaked out, even the people who were HIV positive . . . [BBRT] was mainly for

positive people to meet other positive people . . . I just started the web-site out of frustration with other websites where there was a lot of rejection happening.

(Leahy 2014)

Pigmaster confirms in this interview that his primary aim in founding BBRT was to establish a poz-friendly cruising site in which HIV-positive men could safely sort for casual partners:

[T]here are negative people too though who do come to the website – we have some that put down that they use condoms but they just like our website. [Other] negative people actually have a more informed choice because there is no guessing. They would like to meet people who are undetectable.[13]

As Pigmaster explains, BBRT profiles are specifically designed to inform such choices and support risk reduction practices among its members. By 2014, the prompt for HIV status on BBRT members' profiles offered no fewer than ten response options, including 'Undetectable' and 'Neg + PREP'. These profile specifications enable members to arrange sex without condoms while reduc-ing the risks of HIV transmission associated with any sex that eventuates. They serve as calculative devices that sensitise subjects to the differences that various clinical and pharmaceutical strategies make for HIV prevention. In this respect, BBRT represents a fascinating convergence of digital and clini-cal technologies that institutes and formalises new practices of risk reduction among its members. Indeed, this characteristic of the website leads HIV pre-vention advocate Marc André LeBlanc to criticise the organised HIV sector in Canada for its comparative lack of specificity when it comes to calculating the risk of different sexual practices: 'Let's be honest', he says,

[BBRT's response options are] considerably more nuanced than what we see in most prevention messages and HIV-related studies. . . . Will the HIV prevention field find more nuanced ways to discuss serostatus and the range of risk reduction options that are now available?

(LeBlanc 2014)[14]

Of course, none of these formatting options prevent some BBRT members from 'bug-chasing' or 'gift-giving' – i.e. seeking out partners of different HIV status with some intention of deliberate infection. But tellingly, the world's largest barebacking hookup site does not permit references to such practices on the profile statements of members. As Pigmaster reports, 'We would edit that reference out of their profiles when we see it' (Leahy 2014). This ren-ders the claim that viral transmission operates within this culture as a way of forming 'relations and networks understood in terms of kinship' (Dean 2009, p. 80) tendentious at best. The world's most popular website and extensive digital infrastructure for arranging bareback sex is explicitly designed to encourage sorting practices that reduce the risk of HIV transmission associated with bareback sex.

Conclusion

In this chapter I have situated barebacking – both the practice and the desire – in terms of the scientific and technical infrastructures that produce and attend to it. From this perspective, sex without condoms is multiple. Sometimes it is produced as barebacking. Sometimes it is produced as serosorting; sometimes 'negotiated safety'. Sometimes it is produced as an erotic transgression of gay community and public health and gay norms. At other times it is produced as an innovative HIV prevention practice. How it is enacted is a question that is inseparable from the knowledge practices and technical infrastructures that apprehend and mediate it. From this perspective, sex without condoms is a fitting example of what Annemarie Mol has called 'ontological politics' – a term she coins to describe the active shaping of reality through different techniques and knowledge practices (Mol 2002). That is to say, it is multiply enacted – and realising the concerns of HIV prevention involves attending carefully to the diverse ways and circumstances in which it is enacted without occasioning HIV transmission. Part of this project involves understanding safe sex as a dynamic practice that takes different forms in different historical and cultural contexts (Race 2003). To this end, I have found an analytic distinction between normative morality and practical ethics a useful way of bringing certain innovations in HIV prevention to wider attention.

Notes

1 Some critics pointed to the risk of HIV super-infection, but in the small number of documented cases in which this has occurred, it is rarely found to be clinically relevant (Blackard & Mayer 2004).
2 This piece appears in the mainstream gay publication *The Advocate* and refers to a 1995 editorial in *Steam* magazine, 'Exit the Rubberman', which thematically resembles the passage quoted at length above, though it adopts even more strident tones. I am grateful to the late Eric Rofes for finding me a copy of 'Exit the Rubberman'.
3 Rofes (1998) provides a critically engaged account of this moment in the North American context.
4 I use this term in Foucault's (1977) sense to refer to the process, peculiar to modern societies, of distributing behaviour around a given norm and producing it in terms of normal or abnormal individuality. I want to emphasise the individualising force of this process of subject formation, whereby subjects are led to assess their individuality against norms of HIV prevention (here, the condom code).
5 The byline of the article reads: 'Dating within the HIV positive or negative population has reduced the HIV infection rate in San Francisco. It also allows for an intimacy previously missing'. On ideologies and institutions of intimacy in the neoconservative United States see Berlant and Warner (1998).

6 On the risks and paradoxes of mass abstraction for minority identities see Warner (2002).

7 On sensationalism in mass media see Young (1973).

8 My use of the term 'grid of intelligibility' is informed by the recent work of Judith Butler, who uses it to show how processes of self-reporting and self-understanding are structured by social norms, in particular sex and gender norms. Butler situates the concept in relation to processes of recognition and self-recognition: 'Indeed, if we consider that human bodies are not experienced without recourse to some ideality, some frame for experience itself, and that this is true for the experience of one's own body as it is for experiencing another, and if we accept that that ideality and frame are socially articulated, we can see how it is that embodiment is not thinkable without a relation to a norm, or set of norms' (Butler 2004, p. 28). The value of this approach is that it directs attention to the conditions in which subjecthood and identity are produced. It asks that we examine the interplay of practice and recognition, and see how social norms mediate that process.

9 Interestingly, these explanations were less pertinent for HIV-positive barebackers, among whom only 10 per cent and 7 per cent selected them respectively.

10 This can be theorised in Foucauldian terms as an operation of power that 'applies itself to immediate everyday life which categorises the individual, marks him by his own individuality, attaches him to his own identity, imposes a law of truth on him which he must recognise and which others have to recognise in him', whereby barebackers identify the excitement of sex without condoms as the truth of their identity (Foucault 1982).

11 This figure comprises 60.9 per cent of the HIV+ respondents in the sample and 41.8 per cent of the HIV− respondents, and is inclusive of unprotected sex between men of the same HIV status (which in fact accounts for the majority of instances).

12 Many participants speak of modifying their practice in the direction of safety upon learning of a partner's HIV-negative status, and the study includes accounts of the considerable lengths some men go to when they discover a mistake has been made.

13 As Pigmaster explains in this interview, 'There has been data out for years that suggests that positive guys with undetectable status are a lot safer to bareback with than a supposedly negative person who may have no idea that they have HIV but have a high viral load through not being on medication' (Leahy 2014).

14 LeBlanc's use of BBRT to analyse the prevalence of self-identified PrEP use in Canada suggests that digital cruising sites are coming to be perceived by a small cadre of 'scientifically active' gay HIV advocates as calculative devices that disrupt the monopoly of established HIV research that centres on the means of analytic production.

References

Adam, B. 2005. Constructing the neoliberal sexual actor: Responsibility and care of the self in the discourse of barebackers. *Culture, Health & Sexuality*, 7(4), pp. 333–346.

Berlant, L. & Warner, M. 1998. Sex in public. *Critical Inquiry*, 24, pp. 547–566.

Blackard, J. & Mayer, K. 2004. HIV superinfection in the era of increased sexual risk-taking. *Sexually Transmitted Diseases*, 31(4), pp. 201–204.

Butler, J. 2004. *Undoing Gender.* New York: Routledge.

Crimp, D. 1992. Portraits of people with AIDS. In L. Grossberg, C. Nelson & P. Triechler (eds.) *Cultural Studies.* London/New York: Routledge, pp. 117–133.

Dean, T. 2008. Breeding culture: Barebacking, bugchasing, giftgiving. *The Massachusetts Review,* 49(1/2), pp. 80–94.

Dean, T. 2009. *Unlimited Intimacy: Reflections on the Subculture of Barebacking.* Chicago: University of Chicago Press.

Foucault, M. 1977. *Discipline and Punish.* Trans. A. Sheridan. London: Penguin.

Foucault, M. 1982. The subject and power. In H. Dreyfus & P. Rabinow (eds.) *Michel Foucault: Beyond Structuralism and Hermeneutics.* New York: Harvester Wheatsheaf, pp. 208–226.

Foucault, M. 2011. The gay science. *Critical Inquiry,* 37(3), pp. 385–403.

Grov, C. 2004. 'Make me your death slave': Men who have sex with men and use the internet to intentionally spread HIV. *Deviant Behavior,* 25(4), pp. 329–349.

Halkitis, P. & Parsons, J. 2003. Intentional unsafe sex (barebacking) among HIV-positive gay men who seek sexual partners on the Internet. *AIDS Care,* 15(3), pp. 367–378.

Halkitis, P., Parsons, J. & Wilton, L. 2003. Barebacking among gay and bisexual men in New York City: Explanations for the emergence of intentional unsafe behavior. *Archives of Sexual Behavior,* 32(4), pp. 351–357.

Heredia, C. 12 February 2006. The same sex scene. *San Francisco Chronicle* [online]. Retrieved from http://www.sfgate.com/health/article/THE-SAME-SEX-SCENE-A-Serosorting-Story-Dating-2504382.php [31 January 2017].

Kippax, S. 2002. Negotiated safety agreements among gay men. In A. O'Leary (ed.) *Beyond Condoms: Alternative Approaches to HIV Prevention.* New York: Kluwer/Plenum Press, pp. 1–15.

Leahy, B. 2014. BarebackRT.com – the interview. *PositiveLite.com* [online]. Retrieved from http://www.positivelite.com/component/zoo/item/barebackrtcom-the-interview [26 February 2017].

LeBlanc, M. 2014. PREP pops up on cruising sites. *PositiveLite.com* [online]. Retrieved from http://www.positivelite.com/component/zoo/item/prep-pops-up-on-cruising-sites [1 February 2017].

Mansergh, G., Marks, G., Colfax, G. et al. 2002. 'Barebacking' in a diverse sample of men who have sex with men. *AIDS,* 16(4), pp. 653–659.

Mol, A. 2002. *The Body Multiple.* Durham: Duke University Press.

O'Hara, S. 1997a. *Autopornography: A Memoir of Life in the Lust Lane.* New York: The Haworth Press.

O'Hara, S. 8 July 1997b. Safety First? Risks of sexual intimacy. *The Advocate,* p. 9.

Ong, A. & Collier, S. (eds.) 2005. *Global Assemblages.* Oxford, UK: Blackwell.

Pigmaster. 2008. BarebackRT.com Facebook fan page [online]. Retrieved from https://www.facebook.com/pg/bbrts/about/?ref=page_internal [1 February 2017].

Race, K. 2003. Revaluation of risk among gay men. *AIDS Education & Prevention,* 15(4), pp. 369–381.

Rofes, E. 1998. *Dry Bones Breathe: Gay Men Creating Post-AIDS Identities and Cultures.* Binghamton: Harrington Park Press.

Rosengarten, M., Race, K. & Kippax, S. 2000. *'Touch Wood, Everything Will be Ok': Gay Men's Understandings of Clinical Markers in Sexual Practice.* Sydney: National Centre in HIV Social Research.

Sheon, N. & Crosby, G. 2004. Ambivalent tales of HIV disclosure in San Francisco. *Social Science & Medicine*, 58(11), pp. 2105–2118.

Slavin, S., Richters, J. & Kippax, S. 2004. Understandings of risk among HIV sero-converters in Sydney. *Health, Risk & Society*, 6(1), pp. 39–52.

Tewksbury, R., 2006. 'Click here for HIV': An analysis of Internet-based bug chasers and bug givers. *Deviant Behavior*, 27(4), pp. 379–395.

Tomso, G. 2004. Bug chasing, barebacking, and the risks of care. *Literature & Medicine*, 23(1), pp. 88–111.

Van de Ven, P., Rawstorne, P., Crawford, J. & Kippax, S. 2001. *Facts and Figures: 2000 Male Out Survey.* Sydney: National Centre in HIV Social Research.

Warner, M., 2002. *Publics and Counterpublics.* New York: Zone Books.

Young, J. 1973. The myth of the drug taker in the mass media. In S. Cohen & J. Young (eds.) *The Manufacture of News.* London: Constable, pp. 314–322.

5 Reluctant objects

Pre-exposure prophylaxis and negative sex

'There is a big secret about sex: most people don't like it'. So begins Leo Bersani's infamous essay 'Is the Rectum a Grave?' which first appeared in *AIDS: Cultural Analysis, Cultural Activism*, a collection of essays edited by Douglas Crimp that perhaps more than any other staked out a significant role for cultural analysis in responses to HIV/AIDS (Bersani 1988). Bersani seized the opportunity to speculate about the endemic homophobia that characterised the health crisis, interpreting it as a series of aversion-displacements emanating from widespread and constitutive discomfort about sex. Sex is disturbing because of how it overwhelms the ego structures involved in the psychic organisation of the self. The AIDS crisis created an unprecedented opportunity for the proliferation of aggressive forms of normativity that proffered as their ideological antidote to this disturbance ameliorating visions of benign and proper intimacy.

Since AIDS seemed to dramatise not only metaphorical but also literal associations between sex and death, fears about sex were projected onto the social groups that figured most prominently in the emerging epidemiology of the epidemic, whose sexual receptivity was readily cast in terms of a will to self-destruction. But for Bersani, the association of gay sex with masochistic self-destruction is precisely what imbues it with ethico-political potential, perversely enough. The pleasure that homosexuality takes in shattering masculinised self-mastery through receptive sex is its most politically promising feature, uncompromised as it is by defensive manoeuvres that attempt to smooth over the disruptive aspects of sex. Bersani's essay reverberated widely in queer theory and continues to affect the field in prominent ways. Vestiges of this can be found in several recent key works on the negativity of sex, its political affects and the critical value of the queer more generally (Edelman 2004; Dean 2009; Halberstam 2011; Berlant & Edelman 2013).

Bersani's analysis is relevant for understanding contemporary discourses and experiences of HIV prevention. Aversion to sex functions no less powerfully today as a mobilising vector in personal and ideological responses to HIV as it did in the past. But, brilliant and compelling as Bersani's arguments are, those who have turned to his essay in search of practical strategies for HIV prevention are likely to leave disappointed or at least perplexed.

Bersani acknowledged as much in the context of the sex panic of the late 1990s, when he wondered publicly whether it was possible for gay men to have a debate that is 'not defined by self-destructiveness on the one side and, on the other, a hysterical aversion to sexual pleasure' (cited in Crimp 2004, p. 293). In this rhetorical gesture and other related stances, one is struck by the polarity of the critical alternatives that queer theorists have derived from psychoanalytic theory. Typically, we find ourselves presented with two over-arching alternatives: unleash the critical power of negativity by embracing the self-shattering masochism implicit in sexuality. . . or succumb to your defences and plot your defection to normativity on a continuum that ranges from 'redemptive pastoralism' (Bersani 1988) to 'reproductive futurity' (Edelman 2004). Drawing the battle lines in such stark terms has certainly been productive for queer theory: it has generated exacting analyses that have consolidated the predominance of psychoanalytic critique as a key genre in the field. But it has not got us very far in terms of HIV prevention. Referring to critical perspectives on the appeal of sexual self-immolation, David Halperin suggests, 'I cannot think of *a single concrete or practical proposal* for stopping the epidemic that has been put forward on that basis' (Halperin 2007, p. 101).

The issue here is not merely policy application, which is hardly an ideal measure or final determinant of the value of sexuality scholarship after all. Also at stake are the reductive effects of the habits of interpretation we find in the thesis of sexual negativity. In this culture of thought, the significance of ordinary practices seems to depend on what team the critic assigns them to in a dialectical joust between reproductive hegemony and resistance – an inter-pretative habit that tends to inflate such practices as 'deeply overmeaningful' (Berlant 2007), however mundane, ambiguous, happenstance or multiple they may be in their practical meaning or actual experiencing. In HIV cul-tural analysis this tendency finds its apotheosis in recent work by Tim Dean (2009), which proceeds by clearing the field as far as possible of any inconven-ient empirical variety to pave the way for what emerges as the main game of cultural analysis: a celebration of barebacking, in this instance, for its heroic resistance to homonormative ideals of marriage, reproductive kinship and private coupledom.

Is there some other way to keep hold of the unsettling aspects of sex that does not resolve neatly into the critical alternatives of ideological reproduc-tion or galloping resistance? Can we acknowledge what is confronting about sex without proposing self-annihilation as some sort of heroic political pro-gramme? Is it possible to mobilise the disturbances of sex to think more constructively about HIV prevention, research and education? In this chapter I want to extend Bersani's insights about the perturbations of sex while devel-oping an alternative conceptualisation of the sexual encounter that may alter the terms through which its critical impacts are felt. This involves supple-menting the genre of critique with a style of methodological reflection and experimentation informed by the principles espoused in science and technol-ogy studies and process philosophy—the work of A. N. Whitehead, Isabelle

Stengers, Gilles Deleuze and Bruno Latour, among others. It is my hope that the conceptualisation of the *event* mobilised in this body of work enables a more dynamic and processual approach to encounters than that offered in practices of hegemonic and counterhegemonic determination.

To approach the encounter as an event is to promote active attention to how the coming together of various elements produces material transformations. While event-thinking emerges from a different philosophical tradition than psychoanalytic theory, its attention to what happens when different entities encounter each other in a new way makes it particularly useful for attending to circumstances 'when the organisation of the self is momentarily disturbed by sensations or affective processes somehow "beyond" those connected with psychic organisation' (Bersani 1988, p. 217) – circumstances that are taken to occasion sexual pleasure. Here, psychoanalysis might be situated as one of the most developed (though by no means incontrovertible) accounts of common styles of human prehension, especially those pertaining to sexual experience. But event-thinking resists any sense that prehensions are uniform or determined, or even unique to the human subject. It is instead keenly interested in their practical differentiation and its outcomes, or what Whitehead calls creativity (Whitehead & Sherburne 1981, p. 16). In the first section of this chapter, I set out some of the key tenets of event-thinking that are relevant for my analysis and discuss how these might reframe our approach to sexual and scientific encounters and why this is important for HIV prevention. In my argument, the concept of the event provides a way to approach various domains of everyday life as potential 'sites of intensified encounter with what disorganizes accustomed ways of being', as Lauren Berlant and Lee Edelman have recently characterised sex (2013, p. 11). In this respect, the notion of the event might usefully extend the scope and reach and relevance of queer methods.

Eventful encounters

Minimally defined, an event may be considered the creator of a difference between a before and an after. As Mariam Fraser suggests, 'All those who are touched by an event define and are defined by it' (Fraser 2010, p. 65) – a conception that proposes some rupturing of identity as implicit in any event. In Latour's terms, 'an event has consequences for the historicity of all the ingredients, including nonhumans, that are the circumstances of that experiment' (Latour 1999, p. 306) – a definition that extends ontological transformation beyond the human subject traditionally privileged within psychoanalysis. In an event, not only subjects but also objects acquire new definition in an encounter that entails some disruption of the entities it gathers together.

Grandiose as it may sound, all this talk of human and nonhuman historicity is not necessarily as dramatic as it seems. *What an event is* depends on how it is taken up: an event can be more or less impactful depending on how it reverberates within the range of responses that constitute it as specific occasion. So when Berlant remarks that

> a sex event . . . for instance orgasm seems to make you shatteringly differ-ent than your ego was a minute ago, but in another minute you are likely to be doing something utterly usual, like pissing, whispering, looking away, or walking into the kitchen and opening the refrigerator door
>
> (2011, p. 147)

she is on the same page (albeit of an entirely different book) as philosopher of science Isabelle Stengers, who writes, 'All those who refer to [an event] or invent a way of using it to construct their own position become part of the event's "effects". . . . Only indifference "proves" the limits of the scope of the event' (Stengers 2000, p. 67).

Both of these scholars raise the question of how given entities or circum-stances 'control the degree of unwanted uniqueness engendered in the event' (Berlant 2011, p. 147). As disruptive, disorganising or destructive of accus-tomed ways of being any given event may be, it is only rarely completely earth-shattering – and this would be as true for scientific events as it is for sex. So while some events may be constrained by apprehensions so unbearable that they prompt elaborate defences, other events may seem welcome or even exciting because of the openings and affective possibilities that emerge from them. Event attributions – whether post-hoc recollections, scientific explana-tions, critical reviews, preceding expectations, reaction formations, psychic displacements, particle vibrations or subsequent gestures – are not simply reflective but performative in the sense that they participate in how the event unfolds and contribute to its actualised effects (Patton 2002, pp. 26–8).

The failure of certain events to guarantee impacts that are sufficiently exten-sive or widely felt to be deemed politically desirable or materially effective compels certain ethico-political postures from disciplines as wide-ranging as philosophy, science, cultural studies and political theory—even the pages of sex-advice manuals. 'Philosophy's sole aim is to become worthy of the event, and it is precisely the conceptual persona who counter-effectuates the event', Deleuze declares, in a passage that casts the event as pure potentiality even while it invests philosophy with the task of creating concepts performative enough to make some impact on the event's unfolding (cited in Patton 2002, p. 28). In science studies, Latour is motivated by similar convictions when he takes the surprising step of proposing normative criteria for scientific practice. He values science not just for its truth-value, or for its capacity to confirm what is already known, but for how *interesting* it is, an aspiration that requires practitioners of science to make themselves available to transformation by putting their established categories and procedures at risk. To be interesting, good science requires 'a passionately interested scientist who provides his or her object of study with as many occasions to show interest and to counter his or her questioning through the use of its own categories', according to Latour and the scientists whose work he draws from here (Latour 2004, p. 218). In other words, scientists must be prepared to have their organising categories shattered, albeit in less extreme ways and for different ends than those prescribed in queer psychoanalytic critique.

To replace the terminology of scientific discovery with the concept of the event is to highlight the active part played by nonhuman as well as human elements in ontological transformation. Unlike discoveries, events involve much more than the masterful application of human categories to a passive nature: they involve the coproduction of subjects, objects and other entities. This is of particular significance in the present context, given the constant flooding of HIV prevention with a multitude of new objects, technologies, procedures and devices. Consistent with event-thinking, the nature of these objects – that is, their ontological identity and effects – depends on their articulation with a host of other elements (Savransky & Rosengarten 2016). It becomes impossible, moreover, to reduce the impacts of an event to binary criteria because the event is 'the object of multiple interpretations, but it can also be measured by the very multiplicity of these interpretations', as Stengers argues (2000, pp. 66–7). In other words, an event's character depends on how it reverberates through the manifold gestures, incarnations and responses that constitute its identity. In this respect, event-processes should be evaluated in terms of how they immanently unfold, rather than heroicised or condemned on the basis of some predefined set of (anti-)normative criteria. So where queer psychoanalytic approaches typically present us with two options – self-inflation versus self-shattering – event-thinking enables a more expansive appreciation of the impacts and reverberations of sex among other encounters, offering us a way of grasping their complexity that does not resolve easily into either one of these binarised alternatives. *How to keep events open* is one of the critical imperatives that emerges from this body of scholarship – a priority that raises its own set of political and practical challenges; not least, *how* this openness is to be evaluated and extended in the same moment as the necessary activity of responding pragmatically and effectively to given events based on some assessment of their affects, risks, impacts and possibilities.

In this chapter I want to use this conceptual orientation to grasp recent developments in the field of HIV. A key concern is the emergence of HIV biomedical prevention, which refers to the massive reorganisation of HIV prevention policies and practices that is taking place in international attempts to maximise the preventive effects of medical and pharmaceutical technologies – most notably, the antiretroviral drugs initially used to treat HIV disease. When taken correctly, these drugs reduce the infectivity of HIV-positive individuals, and clinical and policy guidelines now prioritise early detection and treatment of HIV-infected individuals on this basis. This paradigm approaches HIV prevention as a medical and technical problem – a formulation with considerable policy appeal, insofar as it averts the need to confront or publicly address the difficulties of sex.

One exception to this formula has been the case of pre-exposure prophylaxis (PrEP) – a pharmaceutical strategy that involves the use of antiretroviral drugs by HIV-negative individuals for HIV prevention. Despite its proven efficacy as an HIV prevention strategy among men who have sex with men, PrEP has so far emerged as a *reluctant object*, partly because of its putative association with the supposed excesses of unbridled sex. Uptake has been much slower than expected in countries in which it has become available. Indeed, its approval for use in 2012 in the USA sparked bitter debate and a new round of sexual health moralism from gay community-based commentators and HIV specialists (rather than mainstream pundits, as might be expected). The controversy has proliferated rapidly since this chapter was first written and is by no means settled. Its ongoing intensification bears out several key aspects of the argument first developed in its pages.

But this chapter takes the further step of reading these developments as symptomatic of wider problems in prevailing practices of HIV science and policy. Indeed, I want to suggest that a principal (if largely tacit) commitment of the HIV scientific field is to manage and flatten the affective intensities, complications and disturbances of sex. Aversion to sex does not simply influence community attitudes to PrEP (as is evident in the debates briefly mentioned above). This chapter makes the more radical claim that the entire apparatus of HIV clinical and behavioural research – its authoritative procedures, its methodological practices, its evidentiary regimes, its organising conventions, its constitution of objects and its proposed solutions – is shaped by attempts to manage or otherwise avoid the presumptive negativity of sex. Aversion to sex informs the practical labour and professional objectives of even the most disinterested HIV specialists (perhaps especially those). While it is tempting to attribute this aspect of the field to some set of essentialised reactions to sex, the field of science and technology studies might encourage us to see it not as a determined state of affairs but as a situation performed and enacted through existing knowledge practices (Law 2004; Law & Urry 2004). It is the effect, in other words, of given arrangements of scientific practice and the realities they enact.

As has been argued of research methods in general, scientific practices have performative effects – among which PrEP's initial status as a reluctant object could be seen to stand as one exemplary instance. In its carefully cultivated posture of disinterest towards the intensities of sex, HIV science compounds this aversion, producing the sexual as a domain to recoil from rather than actively confront or otherwise embrace in a spirit of engagement. In disregarding sex as anything other than a confounding variable or complicating factor, our capacity to grasp it as a source of knowledge or scene of productively disorganising intensity is diminished. In response to this situation, I want to develop a style of empirical engagement and stylistic experimentation that aims to produce sex not as the fixed object required by the health sciences' practices of prediction and control, but as an everyday source of knowledge events, the indeterminacy and unpredictability of which accounts not only for its risks but also for much of its appeal and motivating potential. The transformations that sex effectuates require attention for the sake of pleasure as much as for science. Attending to them might even expand our appreciation of some important but commonly neglected scientific values such as generosity, curiosity, experimentation, responsibility, mutual engagement, openness, interest and even excitement.

Some inspiration for these connections can be drawn from Bersani's 1988 essay, which can be read for its performative style as much as its substantive argument – that is, not just for what it says but what it *does*. If we pay attention to the manner in which Bersani's essay attends to the wider field of research practices entrusted with the production of authoritative knowledge about HIV/AIDS, we can begin to appreciate new dimensions of the sort of intervention it is making: that is, we can constitute it as an event. 'There is a big secret about sex: most people don't like it', the opening statement claims, only to be followed by an instant act of self-deflation, 'I don't have any statistics to back this up' (1988, p. 197). Bersani's argument proceeds by ramifying the force of his opening remarks in the very same gesture that he discredits their authority by characterising them as the 'rather irresponsibly announced findings of our non-existent poll' (p. 198). From a stylistic perspective this rhetorical strategy may be regarded as archetypically gay: the citation and deflation of inherited conventions is a staple component of various forms of camp humour. What I find interesting about this opening passage is its self-conscious attention to dominant conventions of knowledge practice – an aspect that may be regarded as particularly significant given how rapidly the practices of positivist social science were converging at this moment to determine the scope of official responses to the epidemic. Bersani goes on to dismiss the need for any survey but claims a space for his style of inquiry no less forcefully, since, on his own account, the original claim 'make[s] intelligible a broader spectrum of views about sex and sexuality than perhaps any other single hypothesis' (p. 198). A compelling case is made for speculative inquiry as a critical component in responses to HIV.

Scientific aversion

I have long been struck by the sense in which the evidentiary regimes that prevail in HIV science and policy require participants to disavow their own immersion in sexual cultures and forms of pleasure. It sometimes seems as though the way that one attains professional authority and credibility in the field is by objectifying sexual practice; making it seem predictable; and by talking about it as though it happens somewhere 'over there', among some group of remote but identifiable others. But this gives rise to a problem that the present chapter aims to confront. The very expertise we might hope to cultivate for HIV prevention – expertise in sex as a form of praxis, a source of pedagogy and a potentially motivating encounter – is dissuaded if not actively undermined by some of the epistemic and professional frames that prominently organise responses to HIV. With the emergence of biomedical prevention, it has become possible to sit through entire conferences apparently devoted to HIV prevention in which the sexual and other everyday practices of affected communities are barely mentioned. It is unfair, perhaps, to expect biostatisticians to be ethnographers, and I do not mean this as some sort of professional slur. Rather, the disregard of sexual practice can be considered a function of the regimes of evidence that have come to dominate the field, in which the randomised controlled trial has emerged as the primary basis for making authoritative decisions about preventive action. In this regard, the field is not unlike other domains of epidemiology, public health and clinical research, in which scientists aim to predict the outcomes of given strategies; isolate relations of cause and effect; calculate the risks of specific behaviours; and establish the efficacy of interventions. Such emphasis on prediction and linearisation has been important for health policy, insofar as it guides decisions on the administration of treatment, the distribution of resources and the planning of programmes. More difficult to appreciate from within these regimes of evidence are the ontological transformations associated with everyday encounters, especially those involving sex, drugs and scientific practices.

Given how moral ideologies always threaten to interfere with responses to HIV, the value of this investment in scientific evidence should not be downplayed. It has contributed to the formation of 'rational' public health policy in contexts where conservative assaults on HIV programmes are an everyday occurrence. But the 'definitive' knowledge these scientific practices purport to produce— whether of people or things—is not without other consequence. As Stengers argues (1997, pp. 215–32), when objects are produced and held as fixed in this way, they are not inclined to participate in active or lively ways in the ongoing construction or definition of problems. For a long time, this had been apparent in the field of HIV prevention, insofar as some of the communities most affected by HIV – once considered crucial to the activity of defining the relevant problems and devising effective responses to them – gradually became disengaged from the research and policy process, and were often understood in these terms. This disengagement can be approached as a problem in the performativity of HIV knowledge.

The scientific avoidance of sexual experience and everyday practice is replicated in hallmark pronouncements of global HIV prevention policy. Take the then secretary of state Hillary Clinton's statements in 2011–12 where she outlined the US administration's proposed course towards an 'AIDS-free generation'. The course was said to consist of the use of antiretroviral therapy to prevent mother-to-child transmission, treatment as prevention (in which HIV-positive people are administered antiretroviral treatment as soon as they are infected to prevent onward transmission rather than for strictly clinical purposes) and voluntary medical male circumcision. No mention here of any of the practices through which HIV is actually transmitted (with the exception of perinatal transmission). And no real discussion of the circumstances of key affected populations – men who have sex with men, sex workers, people who inject drugs, transgender individuals and indigenous communities – among whom there exist much higher rates of HIV infection in nearly every country that collects and reports data on such matters.[1]

Part of the appeal of such policy framings must be their promise to address HIV prevention medically, without any mention of awkward topics such as sex, drug use or the gendered, racial, sexual, economic or other disparities that unevenly structure the distribution of infection. And yet, since many of these prevention strategies presume much earlier and more extended periods of engagement with health care services on the part of key affected populations, these disparities will make or break the effectiveness of these strategies. These disparities inform the affective climates in which marginalised subjects locate the capacity to put themselves forward for care or (more typically) find themselves having to avoid it.

The discourse of an AIDS-free generation encourages us to imagine a pristine future untainted by the abjection of HIV/AIDS. With its optimistic invocation of a new generation, one would be hard-pressed to find a more vivid illustration of what Lee Edelman has termed reproductive futurism, in which the 'pervasive invocation of the Child as the emblem of futurity's unquestioned value' compels allegiance to a given social ordering (Edelman 2004, pp. 3–4). Queers are invariably the casualties of such projections, as is evident in their complete omission from this strategic statement. But worse than this, the possibility of queer resistance to such programmes is rendered unthinkable by the persuasive force of reproductive futurism – a realisation that any practitioner who has been inclined to express doubts or even caution about the feasibility of 'ending HIV' in the allocated time frame has found themselves confronting. In the HIV sector, allegiance to this statement of strategic optimism is practically compulsory. Its articulation in this instance institutes a moral hierarchy of HIV prevention options that filters prevention strategies through moral prerogatives to instil them with priority, prominence and fitness for public communication. The prioritisation of men and children as first-line beneficiaries of prevention programmes; the positioning of HIV-positive people as rightful bearers of the moral and pharmaceutical responsibility for HIV transmission; and the persistent appeal to an AIDS-free generation effectively override any in-depth consideration or balanced discussion of the material needs of actually existing adults, not least those living with HIV infection.

Notwithstanding its ideological articulation, some agencies working with key affected populations believe that biomedical prevention offers some strategic and practical advantages for HIV prevention objectives. Indeed, faced with increasing rates of unprotected sex over the last two decades, gay community-based HIV service organisations have been among some of the most enthusiastic proponents of what some dub 'the Prevention Revolution'. While historically, community education and prevention has achieved considerable success, the maintenance of stable rather than decreasing infection rates in some locations has been its most remarkable achievement of late, and the will to interfere with sexual practice has diminished noticeably in recent times or is at best ambivalent among gay community educators. In this context, the introduction of biomedical rather than behavioural HIV prevention strategies bears obvious appeal, prompting organisations to direct the bulk of their recent efforts towards the technical reorganisation of clinical services to maximise access and uptake of HIV testing and treatment. The biopolitical valence of gay sexual behaviour is undergoing significant transformation as a result. Since HIV prevention strategies now take community viral load and not just sexual behaviour as their object of intervention and governance, sexual practice no longer constitutes the exclusive target of HIV prevention initiatives. What is more, the prospect of pharmaceutically mediated viral suppression makes it possible to dislodge gay desires for sex without condoms from their cultural associations with wilful self-destruction. The possibility of safe sex without condoms dismantles the supposed self-evidence of the sex and death equation and it's mapping onto gay sex in particular – an equation on which many queer analyses have been premised.

One new prevention strategy that, despite its biomedical lineage, has thus far been unable to shake its contaminating associations with the apparent negativity of sexual pleasure, however, is PrEP (Figure 5.1). Billed as 'a pill a day to prevent HIV infection', PrEP proposes the prophylactic use of antiretroviral drugs by uninfected individuals to prevent infection with the virus. The US Food and Drug Administration approved the drug Truvada for these purposes in 2012 when international clinical trials demonstrated its efficacy for HIV prevention for both men who have sex with men and transgender women. But this pharmaceutical addition to the prevention repertoire has sparked divisive debate within gay community discourse since the very moment of its inception. Even before it was approved, PrEP became subject to critical campaigns coordinated by large community-based HIV organisations – most prominently the AIDS Healthcare Foundation of Los Angeles, whose president, Michael Weinstein, was quoted as quipping, 'Let's be honest, it's a party drug' (USA Today 2014). The association of PrEP with stereotypes of reckless hedonism has been echoed in popular commentary: the gay commentator David Duran characterised PrEP as 'an excuse to continue to be irresponsible' in a widely circulated *Huffington Post* article that famously dubbed those men 'running to get the prescription' as *Truvada Whores* (Duran 2012).[2] (Tellingly, Duran excluded serodiscordant couples from this titular slur, demonstrating again how romantic coupledom can make otherwise incriminating desires for condom-free intercourse respectable.) In February 2014, Richard Weinmeyer of the American Medical Association's Ethics Group added further institutional clout to these criticisms, claiming the preventive use of Truvada would encourage 'sexual irresponsibility' (USA Today 2014). Indeed, PrEP became so hot in gay community discourse that it brought early AIDS activist Larry Kramer to the pulpit. 'There is something to me cowardly about taking Truvada instead of using a condom', Kramer remarked, accusing PrEP users of 'having rocks in their head' before attributing to the drug a bizarre (but as yet unsubstantiated) side effect: political apathy (Campbell 2014).[3]

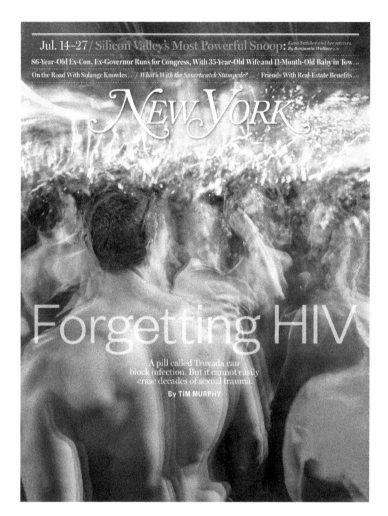

Figure 5.1 Forgetting HIV.
Cover of *New York Magazine*, July 2014. Photograph by Mark Peterson for *New York Magazine*

Apathetic or not, people who find themselves inclined to consider or use PrEP thus find themselves in a highly politicised position, the experience of which has generated some lively and creative counter-responses. The gay pseudonymous writer Jake Sobo took to the blogosphere in 2012 to document his personal experience of PrEP, developing a fascinating genre of public reflection on transformations in sexual experience and risk-subjectivity in the context of pharmaceutical regimes that constitutes a compelling new mode of HIV prevention advocacy and engagement with biomedicine (Sobo 2012). Following Sobo's lead, a number of user-advocates began to speak out against the sexual shaming of PrEP users, with one designing and selling

T-shirts for charity that feature the hashtag #TruvadaWhore, in a gesture of reappropriation that has by now become a stock tactic of queer cultural activism (Glazek 2014). Advocates also took issue with critics' descriptions of sex without condoms on PrEP as 'unsafe sex', and not without justification, since clinical trials suggest a preventive efficacy of up to 99 per cent when PrEP is taken daily. Sex without condoms seems to call for some redefinition in this context. In the midst of this controversy, uptake of PrEP remained remarkably slow, though persistent increases in unprotected sex among US gay men indicated the need for new preventive options. Truvada's manufacturer Gilead reported that only 1,774 people started using the drug for prevention between January 2011 and March 2013, nearly half of whom were women (USA Today 2014). The inertia soon attracted the concern and attention of the highest authorities of US disease control. In a bid to address clinical and community reticence around its prescription, the CDC developed new guidelines in May 2014 that made a point of explicitly recommending Truvada be prescribed to individuals at high risk of HIV infection (McNeil 2014).

The ongoing controversy over PrEP and gay sex speaks to how condoms have served to manage communal anxieties about sexual pleasure and sexual risk in the era of AIDS, providing not only a latex barrier but also symbolic reassurance that gay sex might in some way be made 'safe'. Indeed, the characterisation of PrEP use as 'irresponsible' could only make sense in a world in which the problem that HIV prevention is supposed to address is not simply viral transmission but the moral danger attributed to gay sexual pleasure in general. From this perspective, PrEP commentary is reminiscent of 'the comfortable fantasy that AIDS would spell the end of gay promiscuity, or perhaps gay sex altogether' – an observation Bersani originally made of the hygienic measures proposed in the intensely homophobic climate of the early epidemic (1988, p. 106). Nor is this the first time antiviral medications have provoked anxieties about the moral containment of gay sex. As early as 1997, Douglas Crimp observed that a pervasive and recurring theme in Andrew Sullivan's well-known essay 'When Plagues End' was the 'fear that these new drugs will give gay men the freedom to go back to their old promiscuous habits' (Crimp 2004, p. 287) – a point that appears as applicable to today's otherwise radically transformed present as it was then.

To bring this discussion back to bear on the current organisation of scientific and policy practice, we can begin to derive a number of implications. For all the studied avoidance of the complicatedness of sexual pleasure on the part of biomedical prevention, the early days of PrEP reveal how such aversion may continue to create problems for HIV prevention. If this situation can be approached as an effect of prevailing knowledge practices, as I have suggested above, it is necessary to ask if there are better ways of grasping the risks and pleasures of sex in scientific discourse. This is a practical as much as a conceptual challenge that calls for stylistic and methodological experiments.

The purifying effects of some of the conventions of HIV empirical science have sparked my interest in the use of *anecdote* – that widespread but scientifically degraded form of knowledge relation. Since it moves an incident of private life into broader circulation, we might say that the anecdote creates some degree of interference with the normal compartmentalisation of privacy, publicness, intimacy, knowledge and so forth. I am interested in the anecdote's capacity to produce a form of knowledge that is partial and fragmentary but also intimate and textured.[4] Far from predictable, the anecdote may prompt a form of reflection that is both conditional and speculative. It may be used to provide a partial glimpse into the way that worlds might come together, or fall apart: the unexpected things that can happen. In this respect, it could supply a welcome rejoinder to the rational, intentional subject that has become such a feature of HIV prevention discourse today. To approach private experience as incidental and eventful is to attend more actively and carefully to the contingency of events in their unfolding – and then attempt to circulate this training of the attention. In the anecdote, objects misbehave. Worlds affect events. People do not just act on things, things happen to people – and this could derail some of the force of those accounts steeped in myths of self-mastery.

Mike Michael has riffed on the anecdote as a 'research device' in which an event is not simply reflected but also acted upon; that is, performative (Michael 2012). But Michael is also alive to the sense in which anecdotalisation acts upon us, with its capacity to disturb given relations of knowledge. From this perspective, the anecdote can be approached as a disordering device: an event and source of lived impact from which the identities of the research, researcher and researched newly emerge. In what follows I try to demonstrate the value of thinking – however provisionally – with open intimacy and emphasise the need to be surprised by our encounters, installing this surprise as a methodological principle and starting point (see Latour 2004).

PrEP: initial apprehensions

This chapter began its life as a speculative exercise that emerged from a series of encounters and an overall impression – based on my participation in gay culture – of what I would venture was a surprising state of disengagement with PrEP. PrEP kept emerging as a *reluctant object*: an object that may well make a tangible difference to people's lives, but whose promise is so threatening or confronting to enduring habits of getting by in this world that it provoked aversion, avoidance – even condemnation and moralism. Thinking about gay men's initial engagement (or rather disengagement) with PrEP tells us much about gay men's self-understanding as subjects of risk in historical context. If, for Althusser, interpellation describes the 'hey you!' moment when individuals recognise themselves as subjects of official discourse (Althusser 1970), one way to frame this chapter is as an inquiry into the conditions of *uninterpellation* – those circumstances in which one is led to turn away, to linger in a state of nonconfrontation, to avoid recognising oneself as a subject of risk. The object of PrEP forces us to contend with what scares us, not only about risk but also about sex: how the condom has operated in the citizenship arena, for example, not only as a latex but also a symbolic prophylactic against the apparently terrifying prospect of unbridled homosexuality. Approaching PrEP as a reluctant object – an object that initially failed to engage its intended subjects – may serve as an occasion to rethink the space of the research encounter, to generate new research subjects, objects and forms of relation.

But before proceeding further, some words of qualification are in order. By positioning PrEP as a reluctant object, I do not mean to suggest that it is an unproblematic object or that concerns about it are unfounded. PrEP poses considerable challenges with regard to its effective implementation, use and resourcing, all of which require serious consideration. The issues of nonadherence, risk compensation, cost, access, unwanted toxicity and the possible development of resistant viruses in the context of undetected seroconversion and suboptimal treatment (which is what PrEP would be in these circumstances) are real and must be addressed (see Wainberg 2012; Michael & Rosengarten 2013). (The latter possibility vividly demonstrates how biomedical objects may be ontologically transformed in their encounter with other entities and practices.) But in this chapter I want to bracket these concerns, because they are not the main problems I first encountered when raising the issue of PrEP with HIV-negative sexual partners and friends in casual discussion. At the time of writing, people outside the HIV sector had not even got that far in thinking about PrEP in my experience. Rather, my aim here is to understand the affective reaction with which news of PrEP was often greeted: a reaction of aversion – often powerful aversion and repudiation – among men who are otherwise familiar with, and often have more or less sensible and considered approaches to, the challenges of HIV prevention. Understanding these reactions may be useful for thinking through how health services and educators might present PrEP to relevant publics. It may also help frame HIV prevention as a matter of affective attachments and investments (Gomart & Hennion 1999): that is, how people come to attach themselves to particular objects, practices, devices, positions and identities in their attempts to avoid – or otherwise navigate – the possibility of HIV infection. But the aim of this chapter is not to psychologise HIV-negative gay men, as though PrEP were an object that rational folks cannot but want. This work is motivated by the immense difficulty I have experienced as an HIV-positive man involved in the field not only in thinking about PrEP but also in trying to imagine how things must appear and be experienced by those of different serostatus. Rather than interpret this difficulty as some sort of personal shortcoming, here I install it as a methodological starting point and default presumption: we do not know what is going on for other people, but must presume *not to know* and be prepared to be surprised by our encounters. In other words, my thinking emerges from my own initial reluctance to think about PrEP. . . and then a series of dumb questions.

A few dumb questions

Dumb question number 1: I posted a link on my Facebook page in 2012 to a news piece entitled 'A Game-Changer in the Fight against HIV' (Cahill 2012). The article was a fairly straightforward, well-written account that outlined the findings from PrEP trials and described the prophylactic as a promising strategy. Given how fed up we are thirty years on with the persistence of this epidemic and considering the widespread desire for an end to it, you would think that news like this would attract a little attention. But from among my bevvy of overtly gay Facebook friends, shown posing at gyms and parties and parades, only one person 'liked' it. Even news about what I had for breakfast attracted more attention.

Now it would be foolish to draw any strict conclusions from this flimsy piece of 'data', and there are a number of ways to interpret the findings. Perhaps it was the wrong time of day, or a newsfeed or algorithmic issue, or a problem with my recruitment strategy (my friends are very odd and unrepresentative, after all). Perhaps it was indicative of information overload, or there were other more captivating things going on at the time. Difficult as this line of questioning is to disentangle from the preoccupations of Facebook interaction more generally, these considerations can usefully be brought to any survey, online or otherwise. Data are always mediated by the sociotechnical arrangements that make them available to us, and it is good to get specific about these techniques and mediations. Ever the social researcher, I decided to consult with another expert in this particular medium and asked my boyfriend at the time what this appalling response rate could be about. 'Well, liking it could be taken as an admission of wanting or having unsafe sex', he said, 'something that people are reluctant to identify themselves with in public'.

This interpretation is valuable and interesting, not necessarily because it is representative or definitive in any way, but because it gives us partial insight into some of the conditions of articulation and silence around PrEP. Expressing a personal interest in PrEP involves acknowledging to oneself and to others that one's practices are not as safe as they could or 'ought' to be. This observation can be used to begin to understand the absence of *public* expression of demand for PrEP at the time – an issue that flummoxed many clinical researchers in the area. But it also opens up a series of broader considerations. Engaging personally with PrEP involves confronting oneself, not only as a subject of risk, but as a subject of illicit or socially unsanctioned sex.

Encounter number 2. This exchange occurred after sex with a twenty-five-year-old HIV-negative man at his home. We had used condoms, which were conveniently at hand: the guy was clearly well versed in the practices of arranging safe casual sex. After sex we got into a discussion about our interests and work, and I raised the topic of PrEP. The topic needed some explanation. While he was well educated and seemed to be HIV prevention-savvy and had a vague sense of having heard about something along these lines, he was unclear about the details or of what it might consist. After my explanation, he became quite animated and disturbed: I was surprised at how upset he became. He could not understand why people could not just use condoms. On further discussion it emerged that he had previously been in a one or two-year relationship with an HIV-positive man. Since he had managed to sustain condom use in what he described as challenging circumstances, he believed condoms should be a sufficient strategy.

How can we understand this objection to PrEP and its relation to an attachment to condoms? For Lauren Berlant, an object of attachment can be understood as 'a cluster of promises we want someone or something to make to us and make possible for us' (2011, p. 23). For Berlant, a relation of 'cruel optimism' exists when the loss of that something seems unendurable because 'the continuity of its form provides something of the continuity of the subject's sense of what it means to keep on living and look forward to being in the world' (2011, p. 24). I am not sure that an attachment to condoms is always a relation of *cruel* optimism exactly (not, at least, when condoms are used consistently and effectively), but it is an object of attachment in Berlant's terms, and for many gay men the promise they offer is the promise of protection from HIV infection. This is a hard-wrought attachment – a carefully habituated practice – that involves incorporating the condom into an affectively charged and potentially disorganising scene of intensity. Despite the difficulty of this attachment and the conditions that militate against it, many gay men have managed to install it as a habitual and ongoing practice.

I am interested in the sense in which this habituation might be considered to have staved off the unbearable immediacy of the threat of HIV. Of interest here are the processes through which condom use is transformed from a decisional event into a practice – and a matter of habit. One might have assumed that consistent condom use represents an instance of effective interpellation into HIV prevention discourse. After all, is this not precisely what HIV educators want gay men to do? But in becoming habitual, the condom acquires a form that provides a measure of freedom beyond immediacy, staving off the unsustainable 'decisionism of a life lived minute to minute' – that is, in crisis mentality (Berlant 2011, p. 63). One thing that condoms have been good for, in other words, is avoiding thinking too much – and too intimately – about what at some level is unthinkable, the threat of HIV.[5] If condoms *have* functioned as a way to preserve a mode of ordinariness in a situation of unendurable and ongoing crisis, then this would overturn our usual assumptions about the decisionality of safe sex. In the mode of consistency, we do not *decide* to use condoms. They are used habitually, unthinkingly, and this operates as a source of comfort. The condom habit may in this sense be a way to *exempt* oneself from a repeated and traumatic interpellation by risk discourse. From this perspective, it could be thought to operate as a habitual way of avoiding the question. Of course, there are other mechanisms for doing this – the condom is perhaps least problematic (and also happens to have some beneficial side effects, such as preventing HIV transmission!). Consider the assumption, typical among some of my peers, that *we* are not the intended recipients of these irritating, never-ending messages and campaigns; those *other* evil barebackers/ young gay men/scene queens/sex addicts/(fill in the appropriate 'other') are.

In the context of this attachment to condoms – which is at once often difficult and optimistic – and the emotional energy and investment it involves, PrEP is likely to materialise as both a threatening proposition and a challenging interference.[6] What it threatens is not simply the subject's preferences or convictions with regard to HIV prevention but the sense of continuity that consists in habituated adherence to a particular formal investment in the cluster of promises that is encapsulated in more established prevention objects. From this perspective, the moralism that surrounds PrEP might be understood as a way to counter the threat that a different logic – a different package for delivering on this cluster of promises – poses to this hard-wrought and strenuously maintained attachment.

This is a relevant consideration, I think, for proponents of PrEP, who must find ways to anticipate and respond to this sort of resistance. It is analogous to the resistance first encountered in discussions of 'negotiated safety' that posed a similar sort of threat to investments in the formal structure of safe sex (see my discussion in Chapter 1). One insight that can be drawn from this episode is the challenge implicit in affirming some people's commitment to consistent condom use while presenting and articulating PrEP among those who may need or serve to benefit from it. While some proponents insist that PrEP is not a replacement for condoms but rather a supplement, I do not think that this insistence is realistic. It fails to anticipate how PrEP materialises in practical terms, not only as an option but also as a substitute – and, for some, a source of interference. What it interferes with is the self-evidence of those attachments and associations that have constituted one of the most basic and enduring ontologies of HIV prevention for many gay men, specifically those embodied, formalised and authorised in the principle of 'safe sex'.

To think further about this question of effectively articulating PrEP among those who most stand to benefit from it, my next anecdote raises further questions about how people come to recognise themselves as subjects of risk and possible candidates for PrEP. This encounter involved a discussion over dinner with an HIV-negative friend, a thoughtful, intelligent and frank Sydney resident about my age. We had had discussions before about different experiences of serostatus and sex. Again, I was surprised to find that he had never heard about, or considered, the issue of PrEP. His initial response, when I described it, was marked trepidation and surprise. It struck him as a 'brave new world' proposition that might open the gates to unbridled sex. Not that there is anything prudish or conservative about my friend – quite the contrary, as it happens. But when I asked for clarification in a later communication, he wrote ruefully, 'I can imagine people stocking up on it pre-Mardi Gras and then behaving like cars at a service station all weekend . . . "Fill 'er up!"'.

On this occasion, PrEP raised the spectre of limitless sex and fears of a technologically transformed world – propositions that seem both scary and thrilling, and for this reason can prompt defences. One thing that perplexed my friend most about PrEP was the temporal relation to risk it seemed to represent. Despite – *or perhaps because of* – all the efforts to enlist us as prudent and pre-calculative subjects of health, we are in the habit of accounting for sexual risk-taking after the event, as he went on to observe. The representation implicit in PrEP of risk as *premeditated* is at once more confronting and a different way to identify the self in the vicinity of risk (not to mention *account* for that relation). It relies on the sense of a predictive and intentional subject whose propensity to err is fully present and apprehensible to that subject in advance. This led to a search for comparisons, during which I suggested the contraceptive pill. But my friend rejected the analogy on the grounds that a pregnancy is terminable, whereas HIV is not—or 'not yet'.[7] This line of conversation led into a discussion of his own sexual and risk practices, in which he divulged that he had been taking more risks in the recent past; that it had been difficult to maintain condom use; and that he had surprised even himself with the risks he had been prepared to consider. Situations that might just a year ago have seemed to him unthinkably risky were now situations in which he found himself tempted to participate.

There is a lot that could be said about this conversation, and in many ways it corresponds with other discussions I have had with sexually active gay friends that seem to lend some urgency to the search for new HIV prevention strategies, including PrEP. But for this investigation, the main point I want to make is that, even though upon reflection my friend was concerned about risk, and about his own inclination to take risks (which he perceived as increasing), PrEP was still encountered as a challenging proposition with which he experienced some difficulty engaging. What can we make of this difficulty? What is going on here, and what can we take from this encounter?

The paradox of the planned slipup

I believe that from a certain perspective at this point in the epidemic PrEP emerges as an enigmatic object: the paradox of a planned slipup. It asks us to preempt a possibility that we have become accustomed to accounting for mainly after the event, or as an afterthought. As a proposition, PrEP asks HIV-negative men not only to *acknowledge* but also take systematic, prescribed, coordinated and involved action against a risk that one may not be inclined to acknowledge so readily. Or against a risk that *may* be acknowledged at some level, but that is rationalised as *not much* of a risk – or as something that happens spontaneously, irregularly or in the heat of the moment – perhaps in a bid to protect oneself from the confronting self-interpretation that would consist in understanding one's risk practice as becoming habitual or, indeed, intentional.

It is interesting to contrast this particular orientation to risk with the figure of the barebacker, whose self-identification could be interpreted paradoxically as an ideal instance of interpellation into contemporary risk discourse, as I discussed in Chapter 4. By contrast, the reluctant subject does not locate himself at this address and loiters in a state of nonconfrontation with regard to risk. In a curious sort of way, then, PrEP emerges as the counter-figure of the conundrum that informs some gay men's use of recreational substances to negotiate the pressures of prevention discourse that I described in *Pleasure Consuming Medicine* as 'Exceptional Sex' (Race 2009, pp. 164–90) and the 'Christ-I-was-drunk-last-night' syndrome in Chapter 2 of this book. On such occasions, risk takes on the structure of the exception, in a manner that is at once pre-calculated but disavowed, planned for but not fully acknowledged. Relying on what the popular concept of disinhibition makes available by way of explanation for disapproved behaviours, the subject 'gives himself a chance to swoon' and escape the pressure of the condom imperative (Warner 2000, p. 213).[8] The paradox here is that this notion of disinhibition is a discourse that is largely apprehended in advance. Thus drug use serves as a way of avoiding the charge of intentionality.

By comparison, PrEP asks HIV-negative men to confront the structure of exception head on, as it were: to identify themselves as subjects of risk in the mode of pre-calculation and intentionality. Perhaps, then, PrEP is such a reluctant object partly because it makes explicit something that is difficult to be explicit about from within one of the common orientations to sex and risk among gay men today: the desire to position risk as an *exception* rather than a tendency, a 'straying afield of oneself' rather than something as coherent or culpable as a habit or a pre-calculated decision.

As I said at the start of this chapter, these thoughts are necessarily speculative, partial and incomplete. They turn to sex to query the notion of the sovereign, prudent, intentional subject who is presumed to be always capable of performing risk–benefit calculations in advance (Butler 2005). The affective responses I have described in this chapter should not be seen as essential psychological reactions that precede PrEP and determine responses to it once and forevermore, but should be taken as prehensions: that is, variable ways of grasping things bound up in the actualisation of events (Whitehead & Sherburne, pp. 9–13). Apprehensions of PrEP will change as PrEP enters into various forms of circulation, and it is difficult to predict just what will take place and how. This will depend, in part, on how sex, risk and prevention are enacted by science and other institutional and discursive practices – hence my attention to research methods. A guiding premise of this chapter is that subjects emerge *in relation with* specific objects and the manner of their creation: in other words, subjects and objects are co-produced. This marks out a more active role for research practices than might usually be assumed. For whatever else it is, PrEP is an event: 'All those who are touched by an event define and are defined by it' (Fraser 2010, p. 65); they become part of the event's effects. By querying relations between risk, sex and prevention work, this chapter has sought to participate in this process of eventuation.

One question I hope to develop in Chapter 6 is what to make of refusals of prevention and care, including those I have begun to describe here. This is a matter whose significance is prompted by the recent experience of PrEP but extends well beyond it, for there are broader questions about the reluctance of marginalised subjects to access care that acquire particular significance in the context of biomedical prevention.[9] These questions are not simply psychological but implicate much wider sociomaterial arrangements and attachments: the political production of multiple worlds (Callon & Rabeharisoa 2004). That is, while the line of inquiry I have begun to develop in this essay might seem like just another set of reasons to put PrEP into the 'too hard' basket, on the contrary I believe it represents an opportunity to do the sort of thinking that is needed to address subjects of risk, pleasure, sexuality and HIV in their present complexity. This is a methodological and not simply a conceptual challenge, as I have insisted throughout. I have been testing the value of engaging more openly and attentively in intimate and unsettling encounters, and the way they move our thinking from science to the sex that eventuates.

Notes

1 The exception to this latter claim is sex workers, who (contrary to popular belief) have very low rates of HIV incidence in many of the countries in which their collective activism and advocacy have been resourced.

2 Duran later retracted this argument.

3 Kramer's remarks were reported as follows. 'You're taking a drug that is poison to you, and it has lessened your energy to fight, to get involved, to do anything' (Campbell 2014).

4 Among cultural scholars, Meaghan Morris deploys the anecdote form most astutely, describing it as 'primarily referential [but] oriented futuristically towards the construction of a precise, local and social discursive context. . . . Anecdotes are not expressions of personal experience but allegorical expositions of a model of the way the world can be said to be working' (Morris 1990, p. 15).

5 In a phrase that could aptly describe the outbreak of AIDS and its initial apprehension as a community crisis, Berlant focuses our attention on the 'drama of adjustment to a pervasive atmosphere of unexpected precarity' (2011, p. 62). In these circumstances, Berlant argues, people desperately seek out a habit or a form that might help preserve the energy it would take to live in a heightened state of unbearable immediacy. Adjusting to living with HIV can be described from this perspective as a question of how we 'learn to submit to the passivity and the activity of feeling forced to take on living as a practice, on the way to the deliberate mode becoming a habit, a comfortable gestural rhythm' (Berlant 2011, p. 62).

6 The term *interference* is used by science studies scholars such as Annemarie Mol and John Law to refer to the threat posed by one ontology to another (or multiple others) in the context of ontological multiplicity. For these scholars, the strength and robustness of a particular ontology are always dependent on the various networks, associations, attachments and practices that hold it in place as a stable and enduring reality. Because other networks, associations, attachments and practices always coexist, sometimes in tension, ontologies are said to 'interfere with' one another. But this interference may be more or less antagonistic, serious, consequential or endurable because of circumstances such as proximity or the relative availability of the tension to be ushered into some sort of practical or negotiated coexistence. See generally Mol (2002) and Law (2004).

7 I am not as convinced about this distinction myself, since unwanted pregnancy may sometimes pose a similar crisis of self-viability for women. The similarities and differences between PrEP, the contraceptive pill and their respective historical reception certainly deserve further consideration.
8 Warner describes this as 'the poppers effect'.
9 It is interesting on this count that community-based agencies have sought to de-dramatise the possibility of HIV infection and casual sex to promote regular HIV testing and antiretroviral uptake in the biomedical prevention context. Where for a time there was a tendency to exaggerate the misfortune of HIV infection in the context of new treatments, community educators are much more inclined these days to construct HIV as a manageable illness in their efforts to encourage testing and thus maximise the effectiveness of biomedical prevention.

References

Althusser, L. 1970. *Essays on Ideology*. New York: Verso.
Berlant, L. 2007. Slow death (sovereignty, obesity, lateral agency). *Critical Inquiry*, 33(4), pp. 754–780.
Berlant, L. 2011. *Cruel Optimism*. Durham: Duke University Press.
Berlant, L. & Edelman, L. 2013. *Sex, or the Unbearable*. Durham: Duke University Press.
Bersani, L. 1988. Is the rectum a grave? In D. Crimp (ed.) *AIDS: Cultural Analysis/ Cultural Activism*. Cambridge: MIT Press, pp. 197–222.
Butler, J. 2005. *Giving an Account of Oneself*. New York: Fordham University Press.
Cahill, S. 26 March 2012. A game-changer in the fight against HIV. *The Boston Globe* [online]. Retrieved from http://archive.boston.com/bostonglobe/editorial_opinion/blogs/the_podium/2012/03/a_game-changer_in_the_fight_ag.html [2 February 2017].
Callon, M. & Rabeharisoa, V., 2004. Gino's lesson on humanity: Genetics, mutual entanglements and the sociologist's role. *Economy & Society*, 33(1), pp. 1–27.
Campbell, N. 21 May 2014. Larry Kramer: There's something cowardly about taking Truvada. *Instinct Magazine* [online]. Retrieved from http://instinctmagazine.com/post/larry-kramer-theres-something-cowardly-about-taking-truvada [2 February 2017].
Crimp, D., 2004. *Melancholia and Moralism: Essays on AIDS and Queer Politics*. Cambridge: MIT Press.
Dean, T. 2009. *Unlimited Intimacy: Reflections on the Subculture of barebacking*. Chicago: University of Chicago Press.
Duran, D. 12 November 2012. Truvada whores. *Huffington Post* [online]. Retrieved from http://www.huffingtonpost.com/david-duran/truvada-whores_b_2113588.html [2 February 2017].
Edelman, L. 2004. *No Future: Queer Theory and the Death Drive*. Durham: Duke University Press.
Fraser, M., 2010. Fact, ethics and event. In C. Jensen & K. Rödje (eds.) *Deleuzian Intersections in Science, Technology and Anthropology*. New York and Oxford: Berghahn Books, pp. 57–82.
Glazek, C. 20 May 2014. Why I am a Truvada whore. *Out Magazine* [online]. Retrieved from http://www.out.com/entertainment/popnography/2014/05/20/why-i-am-truvada-whore [2 February 2017].

Gomart, E. & Hennion, A. 1999. A sociology of attachment: Music amateurs, drug users. *The Sociological Review*, 47(S1), pp. 220–247.

Halberstam, J. 2011. *The Queer Art of Failure*. Durham: Duke University Press.

Halperin, D. 2007. *What Do Gay Men Want? An Essay on Sex, Risk, and Subjectivity*. Ann Arbor: University of Michigan Press.

Latour, B. 1999. *Pandora's Hope*. Boston: Harvard University Press.

Latour, B. 2004. How to talk about the body? The normative dimension of science studies. *Body & Society*, 10(2–3), pp. 205–229.

Law, J. 2004. *After Method: Mess in Social Science Research*. London: Routledge.

Law, J. & Urry, J. 2004. Enacting the social. *Economy & Society*, 33(3), pp. 390–410.

McNeil, D. 14 May 2014. Advocating pill, US signals shift to prevent AIDS. *New York Times* [online]. Retrieved from https://www.nytimes.com/2014/05/15/health/advocating-pill-us-signals-shift-to-prevent-aids.html?_r=0 [2 February 2017].

Michael, M. 2012. Anecdote. In C. Lury & N. Wakeford (eds.) *Inventive Methods: The Happening of the Social*. London: Routledge, pp. 25–35.

Michael, M. & Rosengarten, M. 2013. *Innovation and Biomedicine: Ethics, Evidence and Expectation in HIV*. London: Springer.

Mol, A. 2002. *The Body Multiple*. Durham: Duke University Press.

Morris, M. 1990. Banality in cultural studies. In P. Mellencamp (ed.) *Logics of Television*. Bloomington: Indiana University Press, pp. 14–43.

Patton, P. 2002. *Deleuze and the Political*. London: Routledge.

Race, K. 2009. *Pleasure Consuming Medicine*. Durham: Duke University Press.

Savransky, M. & Rosengarten, M. 2016. What is nature capable of? Evidence, ontology and speculative medical humanities. *Medical Humanities*, 42, pp. 166–172.

Sobo, J. 18 October 2012. My life on PrEP: How I learned to stop worrying, and start taking the pill. *Positive Frontiers* [online]. Retrieved from http://betablog.org/my-life-on-prep/ [2 February 2017].

Stengers, I. 1997. *Power and Invention: Situating Science*. Minneapolis: University of Minnesota Press.

Stengers, I. 2000. *The Invention of Modern Science*. Minneapolis: University of Minnesota Press.

USA Today. 6 April 2014. Divide over HIV prevention drug Truvada persists. Retrieved from http://www.usatoday.com/story/news/nation/2014/04/06/gay-men-divided-over-use-of-hiv-prevention-drug/7390879/ [2 February 2017].

Wainberg, M. 2012. Pre-exposure prophylaxis against HIV: Pros and cons. *Retrovirology*, 9(S1), p. 16.

Warner, M. 2000. *The Trouble with Normal*. Cambridge, MA: Harvard University Press.

Whitehead, A.N. & Sherburne, D. 1981. *A Key to Whitehead's Process and Reality*. Chicago: University of Chicago Press.

6   Framing responsibility

Accounting for objects, networks and events

In this chapter I want to develop an argument and conceptual framework for tracking the ways in which responsibility for HIV infection is attributed and the effects of these attributions. My starting point is the claim that responsibility for HIV transmission is always framed in some concrete way, and that these frames have effects that can be attended to. I want to develop a better basis for attending empirically to the production of HIV effects – effects such as HIV transmission, HIV prevention and wellbeing – where these effects are conceived as *events*: that is, the contingent outcomes of the collective activity of a diverse range of actors, both human and nonhuman, including technologies, devices, discourses, scientific practices, health care settings, environments, juridical decisions and desires. Given the complex convergences and tensions between biomedical, technological and regulatory apparatuses that are currently participating in the production of HIV effects, it is necessary to elaborate an analytic approach that might be capable of accounting for more than just the activity and actions of human subjects. As we have seen in the last few chapters, different sociotechnical arrangements make people responsible for HIV prevention in distinctive ways. In this chapter I aim to give more explicit consideration to how nonhuman actors participate in *modes of subjectivation* (Foucault 1990), and to make a connection between modes of subjectivation and what we might term *modes of objectivation*.

Fittingly, the inquiry I pursue in this chapter proceeds from a claim Nietzsche makes in *The Gay Science* (2001 [orig. 1882]) that attributions of causation are always assembled or fabricated through certain forms of technical labour and inference:

> Cause and effect: there is probably never such a duality; in truth a continuum faces us, from which we isolate a few pieces, just as we always perceive a movement only as isolated points, i.e. do not really see but infer. The suddenness with which many effects stand out misleads us; it is suddenness only for us. There is an infinite number of processes that elude us in this second of suddenness.
>
> (2001, p. 113)

To develop this claim in relation to assemblages of HIV prevention, I will first make use of one of the most widely deployed concepts in the contemporary social sciences and humanities: the concept of performativity. Well elaborated in the disparate fields of gender studies and economic sociology, performativity has in recent years become a way of thinking about effects, 'and in particular, to supply an alternative to causal frameworks for thinking about effects' (Butler 2010, p. 147). When Judith Butler says, for example, that gender is performatively constituted, she is calling into question 'whether there is a stable gender in place and intact prior to the expressions and activities that we understand as gendered expressions and activities' (2010, p. 147). Here, performativity serves as a means of countering a certain sort of positivism and essentialism that structures gendered relations and is used to explain gendered effects. Similarly, when Michel Callon talks about the performativity of economics, he is drawing attention to the way in which certain practices of description and measurement, characteristic of the discipline of economics, participate in the making of this thing we call the economy (Callon 2007). On this approach, economics does not simply stand outside the economy, describing and analysing it, but is an important element in the practical making up of the economy. Although Callon writes from a very different disciplinary perspective than Butler, both scholars generate reflection on the effects of certain descriptive, calculative and gestural practices; inviting us to think more pragmatically – and in a less deterministic fashion – about the production of certain ontological effects.

Performativity is associated for some with a certain linguistic emphasis, but this need not be the case. There is now a substantial body of work within the social sciences on the performativity of objects (Cochoy 2010), devices (Callon et al. 2007), research practices (Law 2004) and even scientific instruments (Barad 2003). The concept was also used inventively by the late Eve Kosofsky Sedgwick to think through the social and political workings of affect (Sedgwick 1993). Introduced into cultural studies and the sociology of HIV, the concept may provide a means of reflecting on – and becoming more cognisant of – the *excess* and *constitutive effects* of interventions, whether these interventions are legal, biomedical or methodological. To illustrate this potential, in this chapter I consider recent developments in two of the major institutions that organise our responses to HIV/AIDS, the criminal law and randomised controlled trials. Both these apparatuses have achieved a certain ideological predominance in the organisation of HIV knowledge and intervention globally in recent years; and both can be linked to a certain biomedical individualism, insofar as they institute individual-level factors as overriding concerns at the expense of more systemic and relational analyses. This individualism in turn can be understood to be premised upon what Latour (1993) has called the 'modernist settlement', which separates out human subjects from the devices and technologies that might otherwise be understood to be constitutive of actions, subjects and ethical capacities. Bioethical disciplines can only adequately address this scene of biopolitical production by undergoing a certain critical reframing that is capable of countering such biomedical individualism and its narrow attribution of agency.

The chapter has three parts. In the first I discuss how the criminal law frames responsibility for HIV transmission. Drawing on an emerging body of scholarship and advocacy work, I argue that the criminal law does not transcend the social field, but is immanently involved in its production, including the production of HIV effects. Thus, while the use of criminal provisions to prosecute HIV transmission may seem like a neutral application of moral principles to individual action, it also serves to frame that action *as* individual, to the exclusion of other participants, relations and processes that might otherwise be implicated in HIV prevention. I argue that the best way to grasp the ethics of criminal approaches is to conceive of the law as performative, and to ask what its exercise in specific contexts *does*. Through these means, we are better able to see how the law participates in wider social dynamics, such as the exacerbation of stigma, avoidance of HIV testing, the singling out of infected individuals and the creation of affective climates that paradoxically make it more difficult for HIV-positive people to be open about their status.

In the second part of the chapter I consider the capacity of legal discourse to distribute responsibility for HIV effects beyond the actions of HIV-positive individuals, and to take into account the operation of extended networks of human and nonhuman actors in the materialisation of HIV events. I discuss the case of Primary Health Care (Hall & Wallace 2011) – in which a specific configuration and enactment of medical services was found to play a part in a case of sexual transmission of HIV. I argue that questions of distributed agency and responsibility are pertinent to contemporary scenes of sexual negotiation, where a range of technical knowledges, devices, procedures and assumptions may come into play, ranging from the results of HIV diagnostic and viral load testing to antiretroviral drugs and their actual or presumed preventative effects. A focus on performativity extends the scope of ethical discourse by asking that we take into account the social performances of a whole range of actors, both human and nonhuman, when determining responsibility for HIV events.

In the third section of the chapter I bring this reframing of responsibility (which encompasses more than just human actors) into articulation with questions of biomedical prevention, which see a range of biomedical devices and procedures invested with some potential for HIV prevention. In particular, I focus on the procedures used to evaluate these devices, such as the randomised controlled trial. What is often missing from these procedures is a consideration of *what these devices may do in the world* beyond the frame of evaluation: in other words, their constitutive effects. To some extent, these effects are impossible fully to predict, and herein lies the challenge. This raises the responsibility of those issuing these devices and procedures to engage their users in an ongoing fashion in relation to the question of how these devices and procedures are enacted: a training of the attention that I outline as *responsive attentiveness*.

At one level, this chapter attempts to intervene in the processes through which certain human subjects are made exclusively responsible for the unaccounted effects of biomedical interventions. By drawing on notions of hybrid action developed within the field of science and technology studies, we can build an alternative understanding of public health responsibilities that avoids these disciplinary implications. My argument also diverges from the pre-emptive role that social science often takes on in responses to biomedical developments. Instead, I favour a training of the attention to processes of emergence and the cultivation of relations of ongoing responsiveness. I learned some of these lessons about experimentation and experimental responsiveness as a drug-using, HIV-positive gay man. Experimentation may be deemed necessary for changing a situation, though it may have all sorts of knock-on effects, some of which can be dangerous. But this is no reason for despondency or attempted purification. Addressing these circumstances actually requires us to enter into new, more attentive techniques, relations and experiments in reframing.

Performativity of the law

What I would like to open up initially for consideration is the performativity of the criminal law. This is by no means a new consideration for those concerned with public health in the context of stigmatised and criminalised activities such as homosexuality and drug use, but it does provide a way of situating the law in relation to key health practices such as HIV testing and access to care, as well as a body of social theory that may help to articulate the issues in new ways. Criminal prosecutions for various activities associated with HIV risk – including non-disclosure of status, exposure to HIV and onward transmission – have increased globally in recent years in tandem with biomedical advances in HIV monitoring and treatment (Hoppe 2017). This has included the implementation of criminal legislation in several jurisdictions that creates new offences related to the onward transmission (or potential onward transmission) of HIV.[1] It is not clear why this trend has emerged. It seems that the more identifiable and clinically calculable HIV disease has become at the level of the individual body, the more individual bodies have been rendered responsible for the risk of onward transmission (Race 2001). What is clear is that a complex intermediation exists between biomedical and legal domains which – while differently configured in different contexts – invariably creates new subjects of HIV prevention (Foucault 1990): that is, new ways in which persons become subject to the moral principle of HIV prevention (whether through force of law, through commitment to community, as one whose body is positioned as posing a threat to the public health, as one who might presume to be protected by the law, etc.). These subject positions may or may not be viable, and they may or may not be well adapted to the practical challenges of HIV prevention.

Those concerned with public health in this context have found it necessary to consider the law's effects in relation to a range of social outcomes, such as HIV transmission, access to services, HIV testing practices, drug harm and so on. And they have found it necessary to question criminal approaches on the basis of the effects, or likely counter-effects, on certain socially desirable outcomes. Thus, extensive efforts have been made in recent years – by HIV activists (Bernard 2007; Kidd 2015), researchers (Worth et al. 2005; Weait 2007; Burris & Cameron 2008; Mykhalovskiy et al. 2010) and international agencies such as UNAIDS (UNAIDS 2008) – to identify and communicate internationally the negative public health effects of global trends to criminalise HIV transmission. These efforts seek to force an evaluation of the law on public health grounds – an evaluation that the law appears partially (albeit insufficiently) receptive to.

To ask about the performativity of the law is to ask a series of questions about whether and when the law does what it says, and whether these doings are desirable. Certain statements or enactments of the law might be said to be successful, bringing about the social reality that they name; binding subjects in desired ways. And certain enactments or statements of the law may be seen to *misfire*, producing circumstances in which the law does not quite do what it says, or worse, can be seen to be participating in processes that undermine some of its express aims. J. L. Austin might approach these latter instances of performativity as perlocutionary instances: they do not play out in expected ways (Austin 1975). Tracking what they *do* do is an empirical matter, prompting questions such as: What does the law do, in given conditions and circumstances? What might it do, in foreseeable conditions? How does the law participate in the making of worlds that depart significantly from certain of its express aims? In what conditions is the law, as it is enacted or practised, effective or counterproductive?

To some extent, criminologists have a way of thinking about these things that takes place under the rubric of deterrence. But deterrence is only one of the purposes of criminalisation, legal scholars say. Other purposes include punishment, denunciation, rehabilitation, incapacitation and restitution. Within criminology generally a growing body of work nevertheless attempts to calculate the deterrent effects of criminal sanctions, both generally and specifically (Dölling et al. 2009). These studies represent a desire on the part of legal specialists to *render the law calculable* in terms of its impacts and effects – a desire that might initially appear to provide some ground with HIV prevention specialists. The focus on deterrence in terms of individual behaviour does, however, tend to presume a rational choice actor – the sort of actor that may be difficult to presume in the case of the sexual and/or drug practices most associated with HIV infection. A performative approach, by contrast, would seek to understand how a range of effects (including behaviours) are collectively and interactively produced through the performance and interaction of a diverse range of elements, extending beyond the individual subject, including (but not limited to) the exercise of the law.

Critics of criminalisation have cited a lack of evidence that criminal sanctions effectively deter risk, and they have pointed to a range of potential effects that militate against the wisdom of criminalisation. These include the propensity of criminal sanctions to discourage HIV testing and access to care; to generate mistrust between patients and health service providers; to intensify fear and stigma; to undermine the supportive environment that is needed to stop the spread of HIV; and to endanger infected individuals – especially women in contexts of maximum stigma where they are more likely to be diagnosed first by virtue of their closer engagement with health services such as antenatal testing (UNAIDS 2008). Critics have also pointed to the law's potential to maintain a false sense of security among HIV-negative and untested individuals by framing a shared risk or activity as the sole responsibility of diagnosed (if not infected) individuals.

It is this latter possibility upon which I would like to expand, for it reveals how responsibility for HIV transmission is always framed in some concrete way. By virtue of this framing, certain actors (such as HIV-positive individuals) are rendered culpable for HIV transmission, while certain others (in this instance HIV-negative and untested individuals) are rendered as externalities – that is, considered external to the culpabilities at hand. The manner of this framing not only raises ethical issues with regard to the equitable distribution of responsibility for HIV prevention. It is also performative: it participates in a series of concrete and practical effects. Specifically, it produces HIV-negative and untested individuals as not responsible for HIV transmission, and it may fail to protect them, too, by fostering expectations that the law is efficacious; that HIV-positive individuals will disclose their status in circumstances where much of the evidence suggests that this is generally not likely to be the case, for example (Worth et al. 2005, p. 3).

This framing of responsibility enacts the HIV-negative individual as an ill-equipped or unsuspecting sexual actor – or so research among homosexually active men in the United Kingdom suggests (Dodds 2008).[2] HIV-positive people are framed as the primary agents capable of transmitting HIV or preventing infection while HIV-negative and untested individuals are dissuaded from testing or sustained (somewhat impractically) in the 'practical belief' that the law will protect them and/or that HIV-positive sexual partners will automatically disclose their status. From a certain perspective, this operation of the law might be understood as an instance of effective performativity, in the sense that the law *does* what it says: it renders HIV-positive individuals responsible for HIV transmission. But this rendering (or framing) can be seen to be contrary to the goals of HIV prevention, insofar as it produces sexual risk as an individual rather than shared responsibility, and thus lends itself to other culturally prevalent but characteristically defensive strategies of avoidance, such as the fantasy of HIV-positive predation – 'the evil perpetrator' – as a default explanation for HIV infection.[3] By binding certain social actors, the law unbinds certain other participants from responsibility for HIV prevention. It thus becomes necessary to subject this process to interrogation according to the aims of the legislation, broadly framed; namely, effectuating HIV prevention.

It is worth reflecting here on how the performativity approach proceeds. It evaluates the law as one element in the materialisation of a range of effects that include (but are not reducible to) the general question of deterrence or prevention. If deterrence is concerned mainly with the impact of criminal sanctions on future commissions of the deed, the performative approach treats HIV transmission as an event (or effect) for which a more complex and extended account can be supplied.[4] Of particular significance here are the affective repercussions of the law in relation to certain other significant considerations, such as presentations for HIV testing, the meanings of which change in the context of punitive legislation and other forms of identifying surveillance. The HIV test may come across as detrimental to wellbeing in a context where diagnosis is associated with further stigma and the social positioning effected by criminalisation. Here, the law can be understood to participate in the production of what I described in Chapter 3 as an 'affective climate': a shared context of fear, shame, secrecy, suspicion, rejection and avoidance (or conversely, trust, hope, care, reciprocity and openness) which materially and historically accumulates to make HIV prevention and care practices more (or in this instance, less) possible. There is a name for this concern in the field of health promotion; it is called 'creating a health-enabling environment'. I am suggesting that we need to think more carefully about the production of affective climates of HIV prevention, in ways that move us beyond the tokenism that sometimes infuses the enunciation of important policy goals such as 'reducing stigma'.

Extended responsibility

This argument about the criminal law approaches it as a device that frames responsibility for HIV effects. It suggests the criminal law performs in ways that may inadvertently undermine public health. But what alternatives to this manner of framing exist within the law? In particular, what capacities exist within juridical discourse to conceive the participation of a wider range of actors, both human and nonhuman, in undesirable events such as HIV infection? Key to this suggestion is the argument from science and technology studies that agency cannot be exclusively contained in human beings – or even in the norms, values and discourses that are assumed to animate human behaviour. Action is hybrid, in the sense that it takes place in collectives comprising human beings as well as material and technical devices, texts, objects and so on (Callon 1998; Latour 1993, 2005). Such devices should not be regarded simply as supplementary to pre-existing bodies, minds and their related capacities. They actively shape them, and must in this sense be considered *constitutive* of subjects and actions (Braun & Whatmore 2010).

With its focus on the intentions and behaviour of human subjects presumed sovereign and autonomous, the criminal law tends to evoke a humanist understanding of action. We nevertheless see glimpses of how biomedical devices and technologies might be understood to play a part in the relevant forms of action and cognition, for example in recent disputes over whether the reduction of viral load associated with antiretroviral therapy might mediate criminal culpability for risk activities. In 2008, the Swiss National AIDS Commission formulated the 'Swiss Statement', a document that proposed that for treated patients for whom blood viral load was suppressed for six months, unprotected sex with an informed partner was acceptable (Vernazza et al. 2008). The statement was controversial at the time and generated intense debate internationally. What is less well known is how the statement sought to intervene in prosecution trends for HIV exposure under the Swiss penal code. The original report makes this point explicit, stating that unprotected sex between an HIV-positive individual on antiretroviral treatment and an HIV-negative individual ought not qualify as an attempt to 'propagate a dangerous disease' or 'engender grievous bodily harm' under the provisions of the code. The controversy escalated in 2010 when the Swiss parliament expressly rejected a call from the Swiss National AIDS Commission that it take into account scientific findings on the infectiousness of HIV-positive persons using treatment when enacting criminal legislation. Even in these circumstances, the parliament undertook to maintain the category of negligent exposure, which under the Swiss penal code remains an offence irrespective of HIV transmission.

This controversy can be approached as a 'hot situation', which Michel Callon defines as a situation in which 'everything becomes controversial: the identification of intermediaries and overflows, the distribution of source and target agents, the way effects are measured' and which usually involves 'a wide variety of actors' putting forward 'mutually incompatible descriptions' (Callon 1998, p. 260). In this case, various parties – legislators, scientists, policy-makers, HIV activists – dispute whether the presence of certain technical practices (treatment and viral load testing) alters the risk and thereby the character of the relevant transactions and judgements. It is worth pausing at this point to draw out certain tensions in the general legal reasoning that animates such decisions. While some clinical technologies such as HIV antibody testing are taken to go towards the production of a culpable subject required by the law, certain other technologies – in particular, antiretroviral therapy and viral load testing – are discounted in their ability to mediate the character of the relevant transactions. The law would appear to be selective here in its determination of which technologies can be taken to constitute moral subjects and mediate the effects and intentions of bodies. Where the antibody test gives rise to criminal responsibility, when it comes to viral load testing the law reverts to its default position and dismisses the test's capacity to reconstitute bodies.

And yet within legal discourse there are recent decisions that suggest a greater capacity to account for extended networks of hybrid action in the eventuation of HIV transmission. In a recent Australian case, the question of responsibility for HIV transmission was found to be inseparable from how various technologies and procedures interacted and performed across clinical and everyday domains.[5]

The case concerns a woman who unwittingly infected her partner with HIV (Hall & Wallace 2011). She was the patient of a medical centre, of the sort that is common within contemporary health service provision today: a busy medical centre that receives back-office support and pathology services from a large corporation, Primary Health Services Inc. The woman attended the centre and underwent an HIV antibody test, which was handled by the private corporation. The test was inconclusive, but the recall letter advising urgent retesting was sent to an old address, the reception staff having failed to follow the company's procedure and check the patient's current address. When the woman returned to the medical centre three weeks later to pick up her test results, she was seen by another doctor, her original doctor being unavailable. This doctor pulled up her records on the computer and gave her the 'all clear' for HIV, but had missed a note on the computerised record advising of the patient's need for a repeat test. A week later the woman had unprotected sex with her partner who became infected with HIV. The medical centre doctors admitted liability, then brought this case against Primary Health Care (the pathology service provider) seeking a contribution towards damages.[6]

The case illustrates the extended chain of relations and coordinated action that characterises health care provision today. It reveals the highly contingent mix of practices, procedures, devices, circumstances and occasions of cognition that can make up an instance of HIV transmission. The case provokes anxiety around the extent to which we can be considered responsible for the elaborate forms of coordinated action that constitute everyday practice. Such practice routinely involves participation in complex assemblages of human and nonhuman actors, the components of which are fallible, though their interaction habitually goes unnoticed. It is impossible to account for the circumstances of this case without thinking about the performances of a diverse array of actors: doctors, patients, computer programs, clinical assays, sexual partners, reception procedures, misdirected envelopes, labour conditions in doctors' offices, beliefs, practices and understandings. 'The technicity [of these elements] is such that they can be combined and deployed in relation to countless other elements, gestures, practices and institutions' (Braun & Whatmore 2010, p. xxi). The case reveals the contingency and relative unpredictability of these relations; their eventfulness and their ever-present margin of indeterminacy.

In deciding that the corporation had a duty of care to patients, the case is determining which assemblages of human and nonhuman actors will be considered the agents of HIV infection, with implications for all the other elements involved. Certain actors become implicated in the event of HIV transmission, while certain other actors are framed as externalities, considered external to the circumstances at hand. This framing has implications for future performances of agency and responsibility: it constitutes the subjects of HIV prevention, even as these framings are always available to contestation and overflowing. But the implication of human action with technologies ought not to provoke humanist despair or nostalgia; we have always been technically constituted. Rather, it calls for responsive attentiveness to the practical dynamics in question; the specific arrangements and relations we find ourselves in, which also effectuate our capacities and actions.

Framing effects: the limits of efficacy

So far I have considered the performativity of the law in relation to HIV events. I now want to bring this discussion into more explicit articulation with questions of biomedical prevention, which are currently reconfiguring the field in material ways. This is a pertinent concern, because the issue of who will bear responsibility for the unaccounted effects of these technologies is still active and undecided. 'Biomedical prevention' refers to the use of certain biomedical technologies and procedures for the purposes of HIV prevention, the implementation of which is a key theme of international HIV policy speculation currently. Alongside procedures such as medical male circumcision (which has been found to be partially efficacious as a form of protection against HIV for heterosexual men), biomedical prevention consists mainly of various new applications of antiretroviral therapy: its use among HIV-positive individuals to achieve viral suppression some time before therapeutically indicated (dubbed 'Treatment as Prevention'); among HIV-positive mothers to prevent mother-to-child transmission; among at-risk HIV-negative individuals as a form of PrEP; and as part of topical preparations to be used by HIV-negative individuals during intercourse (topical microbicides, most of which are still under experimental evaluation). These interventions are evaluated in various populations around the world using the procedure of the randomised controlled trial, considered the gold standard of medical evidence. This procedure measures the efficacy of an intervention in a control group over a set time period through a process of random assignment and comparison.

I would like to suggest, however, that the randomised controlled trial is also a framing device. It configures causation and responsibility for HIV effects in certain ways. Typically this framing stops at the body of the individual trial participant, or sometimes the partnered couple, insofar as it is organised around questions of prevention efficacy. This operation is designed to render the pharmaceutical agent an independent variable, the causal activity of which can be evaluated in linear terms. So where the criminal law aims to isolate the human subject in its framing of responsibility for HIV events, the experimental setting attempts to isolate the activity of the nonhuman actant – i.e. the intervention – to draw causal inferences. What is externalised from this frame is the possibility (and actual occurrence) of other effects that follow from the intervention, whether good or bad, predictable or unpredictable. Biomedical interventions are also cultural interventions, and they always participate in knock-on effects and overflowing. Such overflowing could take the form of beneficial effects, such as the increases in HIV awareness and self-efficacy observed among trial participants in some clinical settings. Or it could take the form of less beneficial effects, which concepts such as 'risk compensation', 'disinhibition', 'typical versus ideal adherence rates', 'drug resistance' and 'transmission of drug-resistant virus' attempt to name in an emerging terminology of apprehension. These events are typically produced as externalities: beyond the ambit of clinical research's concern and responsibility. Significantly, they consist not only of possible changes in behaviour, cognition, expectations and modes of interaction, but also the creation of new organic structures such as drug-resistant viral strains that may be difficult to treat with available pharmaceutical agents.

In this respect, the randomised controlled trial is only a partial framing (Michael & Rosengarten 2013; Savransky & Rosengarten 2016). While it stands as a powerful mechanism for isolating the short-term activity of an individual intervention, it can rarely predict what will happen in the real world when the intervention encounters other actors and relations. This is partly because the trial is conducted over a finite period, and the independent variable, the experimental candidate, is often dependent on other factors for its efficacious enactment. But it is also because the effects of interest are pre-specified in the construct of 'efficacy', which represents the measure of the intervention in trial conditions (which are themselves tightly controlled to eliminate other variables). While the construct of efficacy is generally considered necessary for the experiment, it cannot possibly register all the different processes or effects the experiment puts in motion. Yet in policy discourse, efficacy tends to trump all other considerations, instituting some degree of neglect towards the local and material relations that would need to be engaged with to achieve the necessary outcomes, or which might otherwise be affected by the intervention. Some indication of the relevant relations can be taken from a recent report on a sample of patients treated with HAART – itself a 'proven intervention' – in Togo, Lomé (Dagnra et al. 2011). After just one year of treatment, 30 per cent of these patients had experienced virologic failure, and drug-resistant mutations were found in forty-six patients, corresponding to 25 per cent of the patients enrolled in the study.

In health discourse, such events are typically attributed to individual behaviour in the moralised language of noncompliance (Race 2009, pp. 53–4). But in this instance it is clear that these events are not attributable to patient fallibility alone. The authors point to other features of the hybrid collectives through which care is routinely delivered in this setting: inadequate laboratory facilities, lack of virological monitoring, shortage of qualified personnel, unreliable supply systems, inadequate storage (Dagnra et al. 2011). The effects of the drugs are contingent on the relations they enter into, which are always particular, as these circumstances make plain. How should we account for mutations such as these or their likely transmission? How would the experimental ethic differ if responsibility were more extensively configured?

My point is not to denounce the products of randomised controlled trials – many of us wouldn't be here without them. Nor is it to deny the use of antiretroviral medications for prevention purposes: these drugs may offer something that some HIV-negative people, not to mention most HIV-positive people, need for their lives and to prevent illness. Rather, my aim is to open up the question of how best to take account of this wider range of variable effects in the process of their making. Specifically, what research practices, what modes of attention, might be devised to attend to these events-in-process more adequately?

Responsive attentiveness

In the wake of proposals for the biomedical prevention of HIV, a host of research practices have come to the fore. One of these is epidemiological modelling, which sets out to depict what might happen when a range of variables come together, or when interventions are implemented in this way or that. The recent prominence of modelling is interesting because it represents a partial intuition that the findings of efficacy delivered by randomised controlled trials can provide only a limited window onto the real-world activity and implication of drugs. But while these models accrue great power to enact different futures, the models themselves are only as good as the assumptions that inform them, which of course are always social interpretations and political decisions.

Alongside modelling, there is growing interest and investment in the question of how best to implement or operationalise the interventions that randomised controlled trials have endorsed. 'Implementation science' takes a more observational form, with a focus on the rigorous definition and replicability of all the components of an intervention. But alongside this focus on prediction and replicability is another question – how to account for indeterminacy – which is beyond the reach of the population and medical sciences. In their review of the challenges facing HIV biomedical prevention, Nancy Padian and her colleagues come close to acknowledging this point when they advise that 'careful monitoring of what happens in the community when the intervention is scaled up will be essential' (Padian et al. 2008). In the end, though, the research strategies her team proposes have no way of engaging the understandings, meanings and affective responses of the groups most subject to the relevant interventions. Whose monitoring of what happens will be taken into account, and how will this be made to matter? How have the targets of the intervention been engaged in the construction of 'the problem' and its possible solutions; how has their agency been valued? It's this 'what happens' that I'm concerned with, which can never quite be answered by the predictive sciences. It represents the space of collective participation and experimentation we are all responsible for. How can scientific action be reframed to acknowledge and even embrace this indeterminacy?[7] In more theoretical terms, how can we be faithful to the unknowns released into the field of possibility by prevailing regimes of knowledge?[8]

I want to conclude, then, with a proposition for HIV social research that I think these reflections help clarify. Some have argued for greater involvement of social scientists in clinical trial conduct and design, and while I think this is useful and important, it tends to position social science in a predictive and ultimately pre-emptive role, and is not precisely the practice I am advocating here. Rather, I think we need to articulate a new role for HIV social science. We need to devise methods and practices of *responsive attentiveness* to the unpredictable hybrids that will inevitably emerge from this scene of biomedical, social-scientific and corporeal production.[9] This might sound rather abstract, but it will consist of concrete research practices that will be experimented with over time and modified. Responsive attentiveness involves taking an interest in how the practices of medicine and of bodies alter each other in the process of their making and coming together. Just as a body is a different entity in the presence of a pill – bearing different capacities, attributes and possibilities – a pill is a different entity depending on how it is enacted. Neither of these actors (medicine or persons) are fixed or static; they *become with* one another. We must be alive to the range of differences that each is making in and for the other. Responsive attentiveness is different from forms of action based on prediction and predictability that presume to know everything there is to know about a situation to enter it responsibly. And it is different from the civil law notion of a 'duty of care', which attempts to determine what one *should have* known, but in the process gives rise to a general disposition of litigiousness. Responsive attentiveness involves a responsibility to what one cannot know: the risk of being altered by a situation. This also represents a space of possibility: it involves giving oneself over to a shared but indeterminable future; in this case, biomedicine and the law acknowledging (and perhaps even welcoming) their co-implication in the theatre of social interaction, and their necessary responsiveness to it.

Certainly, this means better attention to how interventions are given meaning by their participants and impact upon social relationships (Nguyen et al. 2007). But what is also at stake here is how to intervene in a situation in which end-users become responsibilised for the unaccounted effects of biomedical products through discourses such as that of patient compliance (Race 2009). In the top-heavy world of globalised biomedical prevention, users are not simply configured by technologies (Woolgar 1991), but responsibilised for their efficacious enactment in ways that shift responsibility from biomedical providers to consumers.[10] This is why devising approaches that can better conceive how medical devices and objects actively participate in the shaping of 'human' practice is urgent and essential. To this effect, I have tried to draw attention to the *calculative practices* (Callon, Millo & Muniesa 2007) that constitute the field, which together give rise to such objects and devices. This is to suggest that the same forms of critical scrutiny and engagement to which HIV social researchers subject sexual and risk practices be extended to the practices of medicine and science. The international HIV field is extensively administered (you could say it has reached a point of administrative saturation!). But this administration consists of diverse agencies, which render HIV effects calculable in certain ways. These calculative practices are analysable, they are ontologically consequential and they can always be organised and articulated otherwise: in short, they are performative. How can these different practices and regimes of calculation – randomised controlled trials, observational studies, the practical calculations of affected groups and individuals – be better articulated with one another and more responsively enacted?

Conclusion

The dynamics of HIV transmission are always grasped in some concrete way – by biomedical researchers, population scientists, jurists and legislators, sexual participants, sociologists, psychologists, economists, drug users, epidemiologists, poets.[11] Each of these disciplines consists of concrete practices: *ways of knowing* which can be analysed. These ways of knowing are hierarchically organised: some are given more truth-value than others. The findings of each are consequential, though the practices involved in coming to these findings can always be organised or articulated otherwise. Each discipline inevitably has blind spots, affects and overflowings – they are in this sense 'excessively' consequential. What are the effects of these framings, both alone and in combination? How can we bring them into better articulation to bring an end to the epidemic and provide greater wellbeing among affected populations?

Here I have sketched some possibilities for an extended account of agency, and the attribution of agency, in the field of HIV prevention. These attributions can be studied, and must be studied if we are to take collective responsibility for the ongoing dynamics of HIV. Social scientists and affected individuals are part of this collective, as are our biomedical colleagues, and so are the devices and calculative practices in which we variously engage. The question that emerges from this reformulation of ethical discourse is: how might we account for HIV effects – practically, conceptually, empirically – so that we can better attend to the present epidemic? Keeping this question open is a framing responsibility.

Notes

1 For example, following the creation of the *African Model Law* by the (USAID-funded) Action for West Africa Region group in 2004, thirteen African countries proposed HIV-specific criminal laws and at least seven passed them. A number of countries in Eastern Europe and Central Asia enacted laws that criminalise HIV exposure or transmission over the same period (Bernard 2008).

2 In this survey of UK men who have sex with men, Dodds (2008) found that support for criminal prosecution of HIV transmission was strongly associated with a range of indicators of HIV prevention need, including never having had an HIV test and believing that HIV-positive sexual partners would disclose their status before sex.

3 The legal reproduction of this myth plays out in racialised terms in Western countries, where a disproportionately high number of those charged with HIV transmission offences are heterosexual men of African origins (Persson & Newman 2008; Brotherton 2016).

4 Of course, this is not to suggest that HIV-positive people do not bear some responsibility for HIV prevention, but to question whether the criminal law is an appropriate mechanism for fostering this capacity.

5 The case is a civil law decision rather than a criminal case, which of course involves different jurisdictional aims and principles. Unlike the criminal law, the law of torts is concerned with compensation for actual harm and the distribution of responsibilities rather than the adjudication and punishment of offences against the state. However, my aim here is not to offer legal commentary on different principles of jurisdiction, but to explore some of the instituted rationalities that are currently used to adjudicate questions of responsibility with respect to HIV infection.

6 The court found that Primary Health Care's company had been negligent in its staff's failure to maintain proper records and ordered the company to make a contribution of 40 per cent towards the damages (Hall & Wallace 2011).

7 On indeterminacy as a space of democratic participation and shared futures, see Diprose et al. (2008).

8 For Badiou (2006), enacting fidelity to the event involves performing a 'generic procedure' that in its undecidability is necessarily experimental, and potentially recasts the situation in which being takes place.

9 I adapt this phrase from Donna Haraway (2011) who uses it to refer to the practice of taking care for the unpredicted terrain that emerges from technocultural production.

10 Barry Adam (2011) and Cindy Patton (2011) have each pointed to the disconnect between the technical or population-level analyses that currently underwrite major policy decisions and the practical concerns and insights of affected groups and individuals. Here I am arguing that this technical situation deserves a technical response that may be formulated most effectively in terms of *framing*. As Isabelle Stengers and Olivier Ralet put it, 'It is always possible to maintain that [a given] solution is a solution to a problem that is *technically badly formulated*, that is, to a problem posed according to certain a priori imperatives that have resulted in handing over control to some experts and ignoring others' (Stengers & Ralet 1997, pp. 218–19). In this context, the relevant expert-others are those who contend with the practical realities of HIV infection and HIV prevention in their local environments.

11 See Hoad (2010) on poetry's capacity to register affective responses to HIV prevention and testing campaigns in the context of political and historical subordination.

References

Adam, B. 2011. Epistemic fault lines in biomedical and social approaches to HIV prevention. *Journal of the International AIDS Society*, 14(Suppl 2), pp. 1–9.

Austin, J. L. 1975. *How to Do Things with Words*. Cambridge: Harvard University Press.

Badiou, A. 2006. *Being and Event*. London: Continuum.

Barad, K. 2003. Posthumanist performativity: Toward an understanding of how matter comes to matter. *Signs*, 28(3), pp. 801–831.

Bernard, E. 2007. *Criminal HIV transmission* [online]. Retrieved from http://criminal hivtransmission.blogspot.com.au [3 February 2017].

Bernard, E. 2008. Criminal HIV transmission and exposure laws spreading around the world 'like a virus'. *NAM Aidsmap* [online]. Retrieved from http://www. aidsmap.com/Criminal-HIV-transmission-and-exposure-laws-spreading-around-the-world-like-a-virus/page/1431170/ [3 February 2017].

Braun, B. & Whatmore, S. (eds.) (2010). *Political Matter: Technoscience, Democracy and Public Life.* Minneapolis: University of Minnesota Press.

Brotherton, A. 2016. 'The circumstances in which they come': Refiguring the boundaries of HIV in Australia. *Australian Humanities Review*, 60, p. 44.

Burris, S. & Cameron, E. 2008. The case against criminalization of HIV transmission. *JAMA*, 300, pp. 578–581.

Butler, J. 2010. Performative agency. *Journal of Cultural Economy*, 3(2), pp. 147–161.

Callon, M. 1998. *The Laws of the Markets.* Oxford: Blackwell.

Callon, M. 2007. What does it mean to say that economics is performative? In D. Mackenzie, F. Muniesa & L. Siu (eds.) *Do Economists Make Markets? On the Performativity of Economics.* Princeton: Princeton University Press, pp. 311–357.

Callon, M., Millo, Y. & Muniesa, F. (eds.) 2007. *Market Devices.* Oxford: Blackwell Publishing.

Cochoy, F. 2010. How to build displays that sell: The politics of performativity in American grocery stores. *Journal of Cultural Economy*, 3(2), pp. 299–315.

Dagnra, A., Vidal, N., Mensah, A. et al. 2011. High prevalence of HIV-1 drug resistance among patients on first-line antiretroviral treatment in Lomé, Togo. *Journal of the International AIDS Society*, 14(1), p. 30.

Diprose, R., Stephenson, N., Mills, C. et al. 2008. Governing the future: The paradigm of prudence in political technologies of risk management. *Security Dialogue*, 39(2–3), pp. 267–288.

Dodds, C. 2008. Homosexually active men's views on criminal prosecutions for HIV transmission are related to HIV prevention need. *AIDS Care*, 20(5), pp. 509–514.

Dölling, D., Entorf, H., Hermann, D. & Rupp, T. 2009. Is deterrence effective? Results of a meta-analysis of punishment. *European Journal on Criminal Policy and Research*, 15(1–2), pp. 201–224.

Foucault, M. 1990. *The Use of Pleasure.* Trans. R. Hurley. New York: Vintage Books.

Hall, L. & Wallace, N. 21 May 2011. Healthcare giant must pay $300,000 in HIV test mix-up. *Sydney Morning Herald* [online]. Retrieved from http://www.smh.com. au/national/healthcare-giant-must-pay-300000-in-hiv-test-mixup-20110520-1ewra.html [3 February 2017].

Haraway, D. 2011. Speculative fabulations for technoculture's generations: Taking care of unexpected culture. *Australian Humanities Review*, 50, pp. 95–118.

Hoad, N. 2010. Three poems and a pandemic. In J. Staiger, A. Cvetkovich & A. Reynolds (eds.) *Political Emotions.* London: Routledge, pp. 134–150.

Hoppe, T. 2017. *Punishing Disease.* Berkeley: University of California Press.

Kidd, P. 2015. Repealing section 19A: How we got there. *HIV Justice Network* [online]. Retrieved from http://www.hivjustice.net/repealing-section-19a-how-we-got-there-by-paul-kidd-chair-of-the-hiv-legal-working-group/ [3 February 2017].

Latour, B. 1993. *We Have Never Been Modern.* Cambridge: Harvard University Press.

Latour, B. 2005. *Reassembling the Social.* Oxford: Oxford University Press.

Law, J. 2004. *After Method: Mess in Social Science Research.* New York: Routledge.

Michael, M. & Rosengarten, M. 2013. *Innovation and Biomedicine.* London: Springer.

Mykhalovskiy, E., Betteridge, G., & McLay, D. 2010. *HIV Non-Disclosure and the Criminal Law: Establishing Policy Options for Ontario.* Toronto: Ontario HIV Treatment Network.

Nguyen, V., Ako, C., Niamba, P. et al. 2007. Adherence as therapeutic citizenship: impact of the history of access to antiretroviral drugs on adherence to treatment. *AIDS*, 21(Suppl 5), pp. S31–S35.

Nietzsche, F. 2001 [orig. 1882]. *The Gay Science.* Williams, B. (ed.), Cambridge: Cambridge University Press.

Padian, N.S., Buvé, A., Balkus, J. et al. 2008. Biomedical interventions to prevent HIV infection: Evidence, challenges, and way forward. *The Lancet*, 372(9638), pp. 585–599.

Patton, C. 2011. Rights language and HIV treatment. *Rhetoric Society Quarterly*, 41(3), pp. 1–18.

Persson, A. & Newman, C. 2008. Making monsters: Heterosexuality, crime and race in recent Western media coverage of HIV. *Sociology of Health and Illness*, 30(4), pp. 632–646.

Race, K., 2001. The undetectable crisis: Changing technologies of risk. *Sexualities*, 4(2), pp. 167–189.

Race, K. 2009. *Pleasure Consuming Medicine.* Durham: Duke University Press.

Savransky, M. & Rosengarten, M. 2016. What is nature capable of? Evidence, ontology and speculative medical humanities. *Medical Humanities*, 42, pp. 166–172.

Sedgwick, E. K. 1993. Queer performativity. *GLQ*, 1, pp. 1–16.

Stengers, I. & Ralet, O. 1997. Drugs: Ethical choice or moral consensus. In I. Stengers, *Power and Invention: Situating Science.* Minneapolis, Minnesota University Press, pp. 215–232.

UNAIDS. 2008. *Criminalization of HIV Transmission.* Geneva: UNAIDS.

Vernazza, P., Hirschel, B., Bernasconi, E. & Flepp, M. 2008. Les personnes séropositives ne souffrant d'aucune autre MST et suivant un traitement antirétroviral efficace ne transmettent pas le VIH par voie sexuelle. *Bulletin des Médecins Suisses*, 89(5), pp. 165–169.

Weait, M. 2007. *Intimacy and Responsibility: The Criminalisation of HIV Transmission.* Oxon: Routledge-Cavendish.

Woolgar, S. 1991. Configuring the user: The case of usability trials. In J. Law (ed.) *A Sociology of Monsters.* London: Routledge, pp. 58–99.

Worth, H., Patton, C. & Goldstein, D. 2005. Reckless vectors: The infecting 'other' in HIV/AIDS law. *Sexuality Research and Social Policy*, 2(2), pp. 3–14.

7 Chemsex

A case for gay analysis

In the next two chapters I hope to disrupt normative tendencies within popular discourses of gay men's health and HIV prevention internationally that position HIV prevention as a possibility whose realisation depends on the renunciation of substance use, casual sex in some instances, but especially substance use *for the purposes of* sex.[1] This position already presumes that sex *has* a definite purpose that is not merely self-evident but transparent: a clear purpose – and a sober one at that. Indeed, in recent self-help manuals addressed to gay men experiencing difficulties with sexualised drug use, readers are cautioned against *any* sort of entanglement with digital sex (Fawcett 2015). The capacity of digital media to spark the sexual imagination, engender erotic experiments and invite erotic speculation is not just cause for suspicion in this discourse but constitutes a recipe for disaster and a trap that is said to necessitate complete abstention.

David Fawcett, the author of one such manual, was recently interviewed by HIV advocate Mark King about his advice for gay men trying to recover from drug, alcohol or sex addiction, in a discussion that is indicative of some key commitments of this discourse (King 2015). If readers want to avoid getting caught up in 'a dangerous spiral of compulsive sex and drugs', they are advised in this article to get rid of all their sexual apps and online hookup accounts, change their phone number and other contact information, and give up their favourite porn sites. Next, they should renounce the sexual adventurism or experimentation the authors associate with sex on drugs: 'Maybe you will miss the dark mysteries, groups, and base piggishness of your previous sex life. Get over it, says Fawcett. "It's unsustainable, unhealthy, and ultimately unsatisfying"' (King 2015). Readers are instead advised to *dial up their capacity for intimacy*: explore sex with one person at a time and stay present with them during sex rather than getting 'distracted with some fantasy in your head'. In case there is any confusion, the authors set everything straight: 'Drug-fuelled sex is usually the opposite of emotional or intimate' (King 2015).

Now I would be the first to support practical strategies that actually help people get out of situations that have become endangering for them (whatever works is my philosophy). But the self-righteous, offhand tone with which this discourse dismisses certain sexual possibilities effectively cites with approval normative ideologies of healthy intimacy that have materially eviscerated queer lives (Berlant & Warner 1998; Ahmed 2006; Race 2009), and for this reason it requires critical interrogation. By constructing anything other than virtuous coupling as 'unsustainable, unhealthy and ultimately unsatisfying', not only does this exchange exhibit a derogatory attitude to sexual experimentation (framed as 'the opposite of emotional or intimate'): it also seems oblivious to the sociomaterial sustenance many people derive from sexual friendships. The instruction not only to delete apps but also to change one's phone number and contact details risks compounding social isolation: a debilitating, serious and potentially destructive situation. Meanwhile, the ban on erotic speculation (readers are cautioned not only against watching online porn, but also and even *having sexual fantasies during sex!*) seems intent on ruling out *any* sort of engagement with the virtual life of sex. Indeed, these gay health advocates seem to be agreed on the need to eradicate any such possibilities entirely, in a pre-emptive mission to restore what another writer first described in Chapter 4 as 'an intimacy previously missing' (Heredia 2006).

Make no mistake: what we are dealing with here is the normative prescription of *digital detox*, with the full array of redemptive significations this buzzword has recently amassed.[2] The didactic pursuit of natural intimacy finds its necessary counterpart in recent popular expressions of chemsex discourse, where the combination of sex, drugs and virtual media is said to give rise to horrible monsters – 'the walking dead' (Fairman & Gogarty 2015) – in a frenzy of cultural production that seizes upon the most disturbing casualties of this mix of practices to construct a negative pedagogy with striking exemplary power (on exemplary power, see Race 2009). This has become a disciplinary enterprise of populist proportions in recent years, the undertaking of which would appear to involve dismissing any of the pedagogical activities already circulating within chemsex networks. Such pedagogies grasp the contingent relations that constitute chemsex scenes as potential sources of agency, harm reduction, collective care and transformation. By contrast, the discourses of communal recovery that have come to headline discussions of gay sexual health in many locations produce such approaches as inherently misleading, treacherous and even predatory. This becomes evident in the string of popular exposés of chemsex that have appeared in the UK recently (Strudwick 2016; Fairman & Gogarty 2015) which inadvertently revivify the historical figuration of the homosexual as a menacing predator bent on recruiting the young and innocent into his 'lifestyle', conceived as evil, debauched and utterly over-determined.

The problem with these trends is that HIV prevention and drug harm reduction become aligned with moral compliance to the terms of normative citizenship – something that queer life frequently resists and commonly exceeds. This takes time and energy away from the more pragmatic and difficult work of attending to the cultures within which HIV transmission takes place and in which psychoactive substances are consumed. By finding more generous and expansive registers of response than abstemious prescription, a gay approach to the analysis and pedagogy of chemsex has a much better chance of coming up with ways of reducing harm that resonate with men who have sex on drugs. Though not without their risks, or uniformly taken by all participants, illicit drugs have long been part of the sexual and social practices through which gay social bonds and community have been forged, as I discussed in Chapter 2. These bonds have formed a basis for remarkably effective community responses to HIV in some locations and a number of other innovations in care practice and harm reduction. From this perspective, these discourses of communal purification and recovery promote a disavowal of contexts and practices that may actually be generative of sexual community for some people, and need to be acknowledged and carefully engaged with if the dangers associated with these activities are to be minimised and HIV prevention made more effective. One challenge, then, is to produce analyses of the relevant sexual activities and relations so that the possibilities of care, safety, pleasure and connection that are immanent within these cultures and may reduce the harms of sex on drugs can be affirmed, acknowledged, circulated and cultivated among participants, and multiplied.

Historical configurations of sex on drugs

The matter of concern that constitutes the focus of the next couple of chapters is known as chemsex in the UK, or Party 'n' Play (PnP) in the USA, with both terms being used in Australia (among others, such as 'wired play') to describe the sort of sex the user is seeking, which typically involves the use of particular stimulants to engage in sexual activity, usually in the private home of the host – although smartphones have broadened these spatial possibilities somewhat (Light 2016). Only a subsection of men who have sex with other men engage in these sex and drug activities: about 20 per cent of all gay men interviewed in recent gay community samples in Sydney report having used drugs to enhance sex in the previous six months (Hull at al. 2016), with only half this number reporting having used drugs to engage in group sex (11 per cent). The terminology associated with these practices has passed into everyday gay parlance in ways that are nonetheless suggestive of its sedimentation as a recognisable cultural form. What was once a makeshift set of improvised activities and loose associations has congealed into a legible scenario, a mode of sexual encounter with its own protocols and expectations of participants. Moreover, PnP is continuous with broader cultural framings of sex that circulate within gay culture which have been generative of numerous social possibilities, as I argue in Chapter 8, namely the framing of sex as play.

While terms such as chemsex are deployed most conspicuously today to diagnose gay sexual cultures as pathological, sexualised drug use has a much longer history than some chemsex specialists appear to suggest. While there are references to gay men getting intoxicated to have sex as early as

1933 (Ford & Tyler 1933), by 1969 such experiences were such a familiar part of homosexual experience that they were depicted within everyday gay casual discussion as a deliberate, intelligible practice, as I discussed in Chapter 2 (Crowley 1969). The controversial 1980 film *Cruising* (Friedkin 1980) is also replete with graphic, quasi-ethnographic depictions of the stimulant-enhanced group sex that was known to be a feature of Manhattan's gay leather sex subcultures and underground scenes during the 1970s. (The historical significance of these scenes is largely overlooked by critics who have rightly objected to how opportunistically the film's narrative constructs them as a breeding ground for psychopaths.) Detailed descriptions of stimulant-enhanced gay sex among an altogether preppier and more affluent gay demographic in 1980s London also occur in Alan Hollinghurst's novel *The Line of Beauty* (2005, pp. 385–9). Using drugs in sexual contexts to 'produce very intense pleasure' was clearly also of interest to one of the most important thinkers of the twentieth century, as we learn from interviews with Michel Foucault in which the great philosopher expresses familiarity with the gay and lesbian BDSM subcultures being elaborated in North American urban centres over the 1970s, and considers them to propose that 'the possibility of using our bodies as a possible source of very numerous pleasures is something that is very important' (Foucault 1997, p. 165).

Nor is intoxication for sexual purposes the exclusive province of gay culture: buck's nights, college frat parties and the private spaces of drunken domestic weeknight hetero-sex (and violence) are only the most blatant examples of a mix of practices, the history of which stretches back to Shakespearean times, if the great bard's construction of alcohol effects in *Macbeth* is any indication: 'It provokes the desire, but it takes away the performance' (Shakespeare 2015). Of course, the situation that Shakespeare describes in this passage has changed for practitioners of drunken sex today, whose cis-gendered male

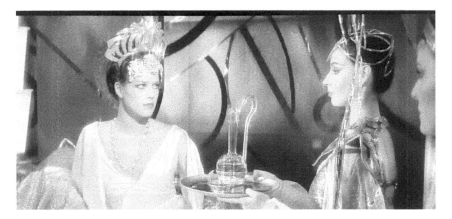

Figure 7.1 Hedonia's potion.
Still from *Flash Gordon*, 1980. Courtesy of the Dino De Laurentiis Company

participants at least have ready access to drugs taken to guarantee 'sexual performance' through normative prescriptions (i.e. erectile dysfunction medications) (Mamo & Fishman 2001; Race 2009).

A more recent reference to using drugs for sex that suggests some familiarity with the practice in mainstream heterosexual culture (and one that never fails to bring me pleasure) occurs in the 1980 film remake of *Flash Gordon* in all its technicolour splendour (Hodges 1980). The heroine, Dale Arden – recently betrothed against her will to Ming the Merciless – is persuaded by the glamorous head concubine of Ming's harem, Hedonia, to drink from a luminescent green potion on the night of her wedding to the evil emperor (Figure 7.1). Ever innocent but nonetheless curious, Dale asks what the liquid is.

> Hedonia: It has no name. Many brave men died to bring it here from the Galaxy of Pleasure . . .
> Dale Arden: Will it make me forget?
> Hedonia: No, but it will make you not mind remembering.
>
> (Hodges 1980)

Ironically, this glowing depiction of heterosexual pre-nuptials on the part of Universal Pictures probably deserves the honour of being recognised as the gayest take on chemsex ever – or at least in living memory. Nietzsche would have approved, I think. After all, the whole point of the doctrine of eternal recurrence, which Nietzsche first set out in *The Gay Science* (2001, pp. 194–5), is to conceive some manner of relating to events – past and present, good and bad – that would make the prospect of repeating them over and over again, *ad infinitum*, bearable. One can only presume this doctrine would apply to events forced upon us (or otherwise enforced) in the form of nasty sex. Such violent, confusing and often traumatising experiences are considered formative of sexual subjects, and are known to persistently haunt the subjects they constitute. But as practitioners of queer S/M sex have together learned, taught others and even found ways of theorising, such disturbing experiences also bear repetition, re-enactment, re-membering and potential overcoming through experiments in erotic enjoyment and what Whitehead refers to as 'novel conceptual feeling' (Whitehead & Sherburne 1981, p. 57).[3]

While the use of intoxicants for sex has a long and illustrious history in both gay and mainstream culture, chemsex specialists differentiate their object from these historical and cultural equivalents by pointing to certain contextual parameters and mediating objects that no doubt make a difference and are said to make gay men's sexualised drug use a particular sort of problem. David Stuart, the manager of the chemsex programme at a leading sexual health clinic in London, has spearheaded efforts to formulate this cluster of activities into an object worthy of government investment and public concern in the UK, and may be regarded on this basis as one of the field's most prominent 'moral entrepreneurs' today (Becker 1963). He defines chemsex as a word invented by gay men and adopted by the gay men's health sector to 'describe a unique sex and drug trend' which he characterises as 'a syndemic of behaviours and circumstances uniquely connected to gay culture' (Stuart 2016). Among these circumstances, he includes a tendency to have a higher number of partners from populations with a higher prevalence of HIV and STIs; issues around sex 'connected to internalised or societal homophobia'; a 'hooking-up culture that emerged from the Smartphone sex-app revolution a decade ago'; and the use of drugs with a 'sexual disinhibiting effect' that he says are 'disproportionately available to gay men via geo-sexual networking Apps' (Stuart 2016).

This formula situates online hookup devices as a definitive feature of chemsex, both as a practice and a problem. But while chemsex has been subject to particularly intense concern, investigation, mobilisation and alarm in the UK in recent times, this mix of activities has a much longer history within HIV prevention discourse and gay sexual cultures around the world that predates the invention of gay smartphone apps and coincides with the growing popularity of online cruising sites among gay men (which, as I mentioned in Chapter 3, reached a tipping point in 2004). Alarm about crystal methamphetamine was evident in urban gay centres such as New York, Miami, San Francisco and Sydney at this time, when the complex problems encountered by many gay users of the drug prompted the ad hoc formation of emergency community groups that went on to produce several disturbing anti-crystal poster campaigns and did a great deal to popularise communal recovery and restorative purification as prominent tropes within international discourses of gay men's sexual health, especially in North America (for a critical discussion, see Race 2009, pp. 164–89).

Chemsex and its correlates – Internet use, crystal meth use and sex with multiple partners – have long been produced in the epidemiological and public health literature as a pathogenic site, mainly because of the statistical correlations researchers have found with HIV transmission (Halkitis, Parsons & Stirratt 2001; Parsons et al. 2007, 2012; Kirby & Thornber-Dunwell 2013a, 2013b; Stuart 2013; Daskalopoulou et al. 2014). As I have discussed elsewhere, the translation of chemsex from a vernacular practice into an object of public health concern has relied predominantly on these associations (Race 2009, pp. 169–74). In London, for example, chemsex programmes only began to attract significant public funding when an association with HIV risk-taking could be shown.[4] A disconnect persists between the public health problematisation of chemsex and the range of problems that have come to matter for heavy users of drugs such as crystal methamphetamine, which extend well beyond HIV transmission (see Race 2009, pp. 172–3). Researchers now acknowledge that men who engage in chemsex do so for a wide range of reasons, including pleasure, fun, sexual experimentation and exploring new sensations (Green & Halkitis 2006; Carnes 2016). But a large body of sociomedical and epidemiological research has found repeat associations between participation in chemsex, sexual risk-taking, HIV infection and traumatic incidents such as childhood sexual abuse, partner violence and mental health disturbances (Stall et al. 2008; Arreola et al. 2008; Hart et al. 2014; Carnes 2016). On the basis of these associations, some experts take HIV risk and sexualised drug use to constitute mutually 'intertwined epidemics' or a syndemic. These associations are difficult to ignore and undeniably concerning (I return to them below). But the terms most available for making sense of such affective problems come from psychiatric discourse, which tends to produce them as the attributes of an aggregate of damaged individuals; pathological victims whose lives are in desperate need of psychiatric attention and normalisation through expert/communal intervention. Little attempt is made within this literature to understand these practices as a culture, or a sociocultural assemblage: that is, a collective, evolving scene of practices, affective relations, meanings, objects and devices with their own organising logics, relative coherence and synergistic dynamics; a material source of pleasure, connection, eroticism, intimacy, experimentation and transformation for many participants, notwithstanding the known dangers (but see Carnes 2016; Race et al. 2016). A gay analysis of chemsex might prompt a further, productive confrontation with one of the central paradoxes of HIV prevention: many of the sites that epidemiologists identify as pathogenic are also key sites for the elaboration of significant social relationships and bonds. In these spaces, participants may be undertaking some of the affective groundwork that generates new possibilities of care, connection, relationality and transformation. Which may not be such a bad thing, especially if ways are found to make these situated experiments safer.

Hookup apps: devices, mediators, genres

As we have seen, chemsex discourse locates geo-social hookup apps as constitutive of the problem, so a more detailed examination of what these devices are and how they work is called for. In the Web 2.0 environment, online cruisers have been prompted to indicate their HIV status among other indications of risk/infectivity on their online profiles, which has instituted new forms of HIV prevention.[5] As we saw in previous chapters, sites such as Manhunt and BBRT routinely make such indications available as mediating categories with pragmatic use, not only for presenting the self but also for formatting sexual searches, and these strategies have been extrapolated to other gay sexual contexts with varying effectiveness. The introduction of 3G smartphones in 2008 extended the digital infrastructure of sex between men in further ways, reconfiguring gay sexual cultures and their terms of engagement yet again. Grindr – a smartphone app designed for gay sexual and social networking – is widely recognised as the first device to make use of the Global Positioning System (GPS) capabilities built into smartphones for the purposes of sexual and social networking. By prioritising geographic proximity and real-time location as structuring principles of cache loading and online profile presentation, Grindr became famous for the impression it gave of 'rapid turnover': that numerous other men were not only easily accessible in any given location but also actively seeking hookups. This was a winning formula in market terms: by 2012, there were 5 million Grindr users worldwide, with 1 million users logging on at least once daily (Woo 2013). It was not long before similar apps emerged to court different sexual taste/identities within gay culture such as Scruff, which became popular among an older, hairier, bear-friendly demographic when it appeared in 2010. But what difference did these new technologies of sexual searching make? What activities and relations did their functions automate? What modes of sexual encounter and communication did these technologies facilitate?

Answering this question calls for attention to the specifics of the user interface. Hookup apps rely for their operations on thumbnail images uploaded by users (or 'selfies'), and these pics largely structure interaction between users. App profiles are much more sparsely populated than their website predecessors and less dense in textual information. On face value, this renders 'browsing' a much more cursory, fleeting, less intensive affair – and face value is paramount on this medium (or torso value, as the case may be). At the same time, the low modality of the user profile on hookup apps makes it much easier for users to change their name, upload new thumbnails to switch profile pics and edit personal details to change their online identity. As a result, app identities tend to chop and change more frequently than website profiles, which maximises the possibility of anonymous use (making them attractive for uses such as peer-to-peer drug dealing – see Thanki & Frederick 2016). Since private messaging bears most of the burden of information exchange on this medium, users enjoy a higher degree of control over the release of self-identifying information, while the expression of HIV prevention-related preferences tends to be differently configured than earlier online cruising interfaces, with few prompting direct HIV disclosure until very recently.

Another key difference concerns issues of portability and accessibility. Unlike websites designed for PC use, hookup apps are continuously accessible via the personal accessory of the smartphone, which tends always to be on hand or within easy reach; users commonly consider having their phone on them an indispensable means of participation in everyday life. This makes online cruising a much more mobile, accessible, reiterative process and ever-present possibility involving gestures such as having a look, checking messages, scrolling, swiping and signalling interest via noncommittal tokens of appreciation such as 'winking' (Grindr) or 'woofing' (Scruff). Such gestures come to punctuate, enhance, distract, enliven, infiltrate, frustrate or otherwise interfere with the mundane rhythms and activities of everyday life. The transition from PCs to portable smartphone interfaces thus reconfigured the 'set and setting' of gay cruising in subtle but significant ways – as well as gay substance use (Zinberg 1986).[6] Matthew Tinkcom puts this point nicely: where the internet 'privatized sexual solicitation by situating users at home while they surfed, Grindr . . . restores the body of the cruising man to the built space of the city [though now with] a substantial database at his disposal' (Tinkcom 2011, p. 711). Meanwhile, the new proximities between data collection and cruising are brilliantly encapsulated in David Caron's quip, 'Sometimes I don't know if I'm cruising or collecting data anymore' (Caron 2014, p. 124) – an ambiguity whose possibilities I mine in further detail in Chapter 8.

While smartphones invested everyday practices of sexual searching with distinctive new gestures, capacities, modes of access and means of arrangement, it was not long before many of the older online cruising sites developed mobile versions. By incorporating GPS capabilities into their software and hardware design, these websites managed to remain competitive in an increasingly crowded sexual marketplace and tend to be used these days interchangeably with hookup apps on a given smartphone, and often concurrently. I will therefore group these digital interfaces together and refer to them collectively as 'online hookup devices' unless specificity is required. Together, these devices constitute a new and evolving *infrastructure of the sexual encounter*, a phrase I use to draw attention to the material specificity of these devices, as well as to prompt questions about *who* these infrastructures service and how, and to emphasise the point that they mediate the sexual encounter in certain ways; making certain activities, relations and practices possible while destabilising or rendering others redundant.[7]

There are of course many different ways of using online hookup devices, not to mention motivations for use. While the default *modus operandi* presumed of hookup app users is the desire for no-strings encounters, these devices are available for a wider range of uses ('finding a boyfriend', 'dates and mates', 'just chat' and 'having a look'). Whatever the motivation for use, these devices nonetheless configure and discipline their users in certain ways: as with any technology, a sense of the ideal user informs their design, and users have to find some way of negotiating this ideal in the process of learning how to use them (Woolgar 1991). This is not to suggest these devices *determine* the practices and experiences that emerge from them. But it is difficult to understand the shape of sexual cultures between men in the present – their contours, conventions, characteristic sequences of activity, modes of interaction and affective forms – without getting specific about the formats, features, functions and affordances of online hookup devices.[8]

There is no question these devices have promoted and consolidated masculinist and racialised forms of sexual capital within gay sexual culture (Raj 2011), although minoritised racial or gender identity does not in itself preclude participation, or operate as a meaningful selection criterion for everyone that uses these devices to conduct sexual searches. Though not my principal focus here, discrimination between users on the basis of race and other prejudicial criteria is an all too common experience of these sexual media. Where earlier gay cruising sites itemised race and ethnicity as active categories for sexual searching and/or blocking communication, hookup apps make these categories matter in new ways by adopting different configurative options. As active mediators of sexual encounters, online hookup devices have nevertheless changed the terms and conditions through which abstractions such as 'race' have come to matter in gay sexual cultures. The appeal these devices make to commoditised logics and the narrow terms according to which members are obliged to categorise and present themselves are no doubt implicated in this situation and have been a source of significant criticism, particularly in terms of how they privilege certain body types (Light et al. 2008). While hookup apps are organised primarily around the consumption and production of visual data, which obviously prioritises certain member attributes and neglects others, their interfaces have auditory, haptic and touchscreen dimensions. One can only hope that tactile and olfactory design initiatives within the field of Human-Computer Interaction get a move on and add a bit of multi-sensory texture and richness to app-mediated 'first impressions'. I await the scratch 'n' sniff upgrade with bated breath – perhaps in the form of a plug-in attachment to Scruff's 'woof' button?

As we can see from this brief consideration of app interfaces and functions, mobile devices have introduced a range of new manners of relating to others and automated a range of new socio-sexual habits that reconfigure male-to-male sexual cultures and transform sexual subjectivities in subtle but material ways. There is a long and rich history of cruising practices in gay urban centres, to be sure (Bech 1997; Delany 1999). Indeed, these histories inform many of the design features and uses of online hookup devices. But any account that represents this sexual infrastructure as just 'the latest version of cruising' misses something important about the specificity of the sociotechnical arrangements that shape its contours and conventional forms. The distinction Latour makes between mediators and intermediaries may be helpful here. Where *intermediaries* transport meanings without transformation, *mediators* 'transform, translate, distort and modify the meaning or the elements they are supposed to carry'; thus their specificity 'has to be taken into account every time' (2005, p. 39). In other words, online hookup devices are not inert vessels or pathways for the same old meanings and interactions. They are not intermediaries, merely reproducing pre-existent characteristics of sexual cultures and practices. Rather, they act as *mediators*: active ingredients that modify the practices and encounters they enable in novel, specifically impactful ways. Gay cruising is taking new forms, assuming new genres and proceeding through new avenues in its encounter with digital media. *Something is happening here*: new sexual cultures are emerging, their self-technologies transforming. We are faced with a significant transformation in genres of sexual interaction and practices of sexual association and community that requires acknowledgement, understanding and development.

My reference to the concept of genre is meant to suggest that, however variable and idiosyncratic they may appear, digitally arranged encounters proceed according to certain conventions that shape and constrain the forms they typically take. That is to say, online interactions are characterised by certain formal features that offer frameworks for constructing meaning and value (Frow 2006). In cultural theory, the term genre typically refers to types of texts and speech, and this makes it useful for making sense of many of the activities I will go on to discuss. Digital media give a textual materiality to interactions that might otherwise be conducted verbally (and often non-verbally). Indeed, it is precisely the materialisation of these interactions *in* and *as* text that invests this scene with many of its most significant and novel affordances, as I explore in Chapter 8. But genre as it is conventionally theorised encounters some friction when set loose within this mix of technical, pragmatic, signifying, interactive, mobile, mediated, affective functions that together constitute the hookup app. This presents an opportunity for conceptual renovation: in genre theory, material or technological elements tend to be bracketed in favour of a focus on discursive processes.[9] But as we shall see, it is the very materiality of written texts and digital images that generates certain new capacities, experiences and affective vectors for app users. Genre might be used to refer to more than merely discursive systems; it can be applied to practical manners of grasping and relating to the world – which are frequently mediated by particular techniques, objects, material conditions and terms of engagement. From this perspective, digital devices represent an opportunity to push genre theory towards a more explicit acknowledgement of the *agency* of material objects and devices in communicative action (Hawkins et al. 2015, pp. 82–5).

Making chemsex public: 'it's a horror story'

In their remarkable collection *Making Things Public*, Latour and Weibel (2005) draw attention to the various technologies, interfaces, platforms, sociomaterial assemblages and mediations that people have used historically to make 'matters of concern' public. This volume curates an extraordinary range of examples of how things have been made public in different times and places which the editors collect together to propose a series of pragmatic questions: *how* do particular mediating techniques engage the relevant parties? How do they bring in the relevant issues? What changes do these practices make to people's attachments to the thing in question? And how is the thing that constitutes the matter of concern transformed in the process?

Chemsex is nothing if not a matter of concern, with various actors gathering around it: chemsex participants, their friends, lovers, families, carers and communities, social workers, clinicians, community educators, journalists, harm reduction advocates, public health specialists, the police, emergency staff, pornographers, critics, documentarians, etc. But the process of making chemsex public is fraught with challenges and perils and might be considered a dangerous experiment in itself. As we saw in Chapter 4, the process of making illicit or disapproved corporeal activities intelligible to mainstream publics tends to misrecognise, distort or ignore the practical ethics that inform and sustain participants in subcultural activities. This is particularly true of the journalistic genres that constitute mass media, because the audience of these media are presumed to subscribe to what Jock Young once characterised as the consensual morality of bourgeois society (1973): family values, hard work and deferred gratification (i.e. heteronormative labour and being a good capitalist subject). In this consensual framework, pleasures that do not emerge as the just reward for hard work and hetero-gendered labour must be presented as false, or narratively constructed as 'getting what is coming to them' (Race 2009, pp. 157–63). But this critique of mass media should not be taken to suggest the scientific genres of socio-medical research are less implicated in the problem. Indeed, scientists can sometimes be less thoughtful about how to handle the ethical and practical challenge of making their findings intelligible and available to relevant pub-lic agencies, since they are constrained mainly by the disciplinary standards attributed to colleagues (who are often presumed to share conservative values) and the peers who anonymously review and endorse their analyses, all the while protected by the presuppositions of positivist science, with all the privi-lege and authority of 'neutral objectivity' that goes with these. Indeed, one only need take a quick flip through recent discussions of chemsex in medical journals such as *The Lancet* to recognise many of the same tropes and ampli-fications of affect that I will go on to discuss in relation to popular media discourses of chemsex (Kirby & Thornber-Dunwell 2013a, 2013b).

As mentioned earlier, health advocates have confronted considerable obstacles in their efforts to make chemsex public in a way that would attract governmental concern and public investment.[10] No sooner had they done so, and no sooner had the topic begun to attract the sort of attention needed to secure public funding for appropriately tailored services in the UK, than it was pounced upon by a pair of heterosexual filmmakers who seized the opportunity to make a documentary about the issue in the ever-popular crowd-pleasing genre of the sensationalist exposé. Vice Productions' *Chemsex* (Gogarty & Fairman 2015) sets out to investigate what it describes as a 'hidden healthcare emergency' in London, billing itself with the tagline, 'it's a horror story' – an epitaph I believe to be particularly apt (though probably not for the same rea-sons as the documentary's publicists). *Chemsex* deploys the spectacle of illicit drug use and non-normative gay sex to incite intrigue, excitement, horror and disgust among the audience it addresses (gay and mainstream viewers).[11] In this respect, it follows in the footsteps of *Cruising* (Friedkin 1980), the controversial crime thriller set in the dark subcultural spaces of Manhattan's gay leather scene in the 1970s, a fiction that can be situated as the documen-tary's formulaic progenitor and closest generic precedent. But unlike *Cruising*, *Chemsex* engages its audiences in the much more respectable register of liberal concern, paternalistic affect and therapeutic sympathy. The film opens with a wide shot of central London, rendered distinctively gothic by the eerie light of a full moon. The camera homes in slowly on a sparsely furnished apartment where a young man sits injecting drugs into his forearm, apparently alone (but actually with the film-crew). Within seconds, the audience is instantly confronted with the spectacle of compulsive gay male sexual desire: the man is sent into intense throes of wide-eyed erotic euphoria: 'See, now all I want to do is get fucked . . . it's crazy', he says, grabbing his crotch absent-mindedly. 'Cock, cock, cock, cock, cock. . .' he utters, apparently compulsively. As the opening credits roll, an anonymous (presumably gay) man offers the following reflections of chemsexers in voiceover: 'They just look possessed: Wild, hungry and desperate. I'm scared of this kind of perversion of the gay scene. It's pathological. There's something scary happening'. The tone is set: we've come to see a zombie film.

Unsurprisingly (given the requirements of this genre), it is the dangerous and destructive end of the spectrum of gay men's drug use that the documentary takes as its principal focus, which it combines with the explicit spectacle of gay fetish activities and non-normative sex for maximum sensationalist effect. Not long into the film, we are introduced to guys who inject in a single hit an amount of crystal methamphetamine that might last many of their peers several weekends. We hear from numerous men whose lives have been torn apart by drug dependence and various tragic circumstances; but rarely anyone who has occasionally or regularly enjoyed chemsex drugs over the long term and leads a relatively fulfilling, happy, but otherwise unexceptional life – a large proportion of users, research suggests (Degenhardt et al. 2008; Quinn et al. 2013). At the narrative turning point we are treated to unsettling footage of a man, most likely suffering from pre-existing mental health problems, in the midst of a crystal meth psychosis, who the filmmakers see fit to interview as he attempts to find a vein good enough for injection, but repeatedly fails to do so, so frequently is he distracted by twitches and spasms of paranoid anxiety. Things get messy quickly and – needless to say – the overall picture is not pretty. For those unfamiliar with gay fetish scenes, the confronting nature of such footage would no doubt be compounded by the film's graphic depiction throughout of group sex between mean, leather sex and kink. For viewers less fazed by such activities, the main source of astonishment is surely the participants' openness to straight documentarians filming them in the midst of such intense, erotic and highly stigmatised activities. But when high on psychoactive stimulants, people may become prepared to do a lot of things they might normally be reticent about, as the whole production of *Chemsex* amply illustrates.

To its credit, the film manages to convey some of the complexities of gay sex in the era of HIV, constructing its participants (and gay men by and large) as still in the midst of processing the traumatic effects of the HIV epidemic, with its manifold impacts on sexual desires, identities and intimate attachments. For some men filmed, drugs seem to provide the most readily available solution to the age-old problem, 'how to have sex in an epidemic' (Berkowitz 1983),[12] insofar as they enable some degree of 'cognitive disengagement' from the anxieties and frustrations they associate with having sex in the shadow of HIV (McKirnan, Ostrow & Hope 1996). The film also conveys some of the difficulties of fostering intimate or effective relationships when the process of arranging sex is divorced from other social contexts, as it can be with online hookup devices, and the dangerous social isolation some men experience as a consequence.

Hookup apps are further problematised for making powerful stimulants more available and accessible, and encounters with practices such as injecting more common. But *Chemsex* fails to verify the prevalence of such practices, which is found to be much smaller than the impression given by the film of an epidemic engulfing the gay scene and sweeping London (Hickson et al. 2016; Melendez-Torres et al. 2016).[13] Nor does the film consider that hookup apps might simply have magnified the impression of a wide and growing prevalence within gay circles by making some men's quests for sex on drugs much more visible (when they would otherwise be conducted more covertly). As I mentioned earlier, hookup apps are also mediating devices that prioritise proximity and visibility. What once took place in venues whose location was discreet but easily discoverable through word-of-mouth to those who wanted to participate now pops up in the GPS catchment area of any given hookup app in any given location to confront the unsuspecting user. Recent research appears to confirm this possibility by finding 'clearly . . . exaggerated beliefs about the ubiquity of chemsex' among gay men in South London (Ahmed at al. 2016). The film does little to temper such exaggerations. In the narrative set-up, an expert informant introduces the topic in the following terms:

> In my day, you'd get asked out in a bar perhaps. These days, [at age] 15 [or] 16 you leave your home in Hertfordshire, you come into London to find your gay life, and you find Grindr. And within perhaps four conversations you're going to be introduced to chems. Within eight conversations on Grindr you're going to be introduced to injecting, or slamming as it's called.

Here, hookup apps are centrally implicated in what becomes problematised as a new sense of accessibility – of sex, drugs and more extreme modes of self-administration such as injecting. But it bears remembering that encountering something by seeing it or having it presented to you online is not quite the same thing as doing it. While perceptions of social norms and drug accessibility are certainly not immaterial concerns, insofar as they may contribute to the normalisation of certain practices, technically the documentary itself is no less guilty than the media devices it frets about of 'introducing' uninitiated audiences to chemsex.

The figure of the innocent, wholesome youth – imminently vulnerable to the corrupting devices of toxic homosexual predators – looms large in this discourse. These figures have taken on a life of their own in more recent instances of chemsex discourse in the UK. Hot on the heels of *Chemsex* (2015), a recent article takes such figures to their logical extreme. 'This is what chemsex is doing to gay men: Inside the dark, dangerous world of chemsex' trades in forms, figures and affective dynamics similar to the documentary, as one might surmise from its captivating title (Strudwick 2016). The article is uniquely placed to provide insight into what these particular ways of 'making chemsex public' are producing on this basis.

Strudwick uses the recent criminal conviction of a London man for doping, raping and murdering four young men he met online to paint a terrifying picture of London's chemsex scene, which he depicts as a macabre, mysterious underworld teeming with deceptive characters, systemic abuse, kinky sex, unspeakable dangers and horrifying incidents. The report is constructed on the basis of a handful of anonymous informants who provide 'first-hand' anecdotes of unseemly circumstances and experiences – including seeing people overdose and get sexually assaulted; tales of people getting drugged against their knowledge or their will; 'hearing stories' of mishandled drug deaths ('I've heard stories of guys being thrown out the flat into a bin outside and being left to die'); people losing their minds, belongings, jobs, dignity and reputation, and becoming sex workers. Strudwick constructs London's chemsex scene as a world populated by two main figures: the vulnerable and misguided youngster with no agency whatsoever, and the evil old predator suspected capable of heinous crimes including duplicity, negligence, sexual assault, inflicting grievous bodily harm, coaxing youngsters into prostitution, deliberate HIV infection, rape and murder. While these stories and allegations are undoubtedly disturbing and require investigation and further verification, the article's fascination with innuendo, mysterious circumstances, morbidity, obscurity and macabre characters means it reads less like a piece of serious journalism than a full-blown gothic horror fiction, steeped in the 'pleasing sort of terror' said to be characteristic of this genre. Meanwhile, the idea that chemsex participants might have any sort of agency available to them other than the digital alternatives of *on* or *off* – *one* or *zero* – is virtually inconceivable on this account, so determined is Strudwick to equate 'one' (positive agency) with criminal intentionality, and being high on drugs with total helplessness: 'In this scenario, every notion of personal agency is removed', he writes at one point.

Drugs are constructed in Strudwick's article in conventional terms as 'powerful disinhibitors' – switch-triggers capable of removing 'not only inhibitions but . . . human kindness', only to replace it with a 'frenzy . . . of accelerating sexual desire, energy, and, often, aggression' (Strudwick 2016). This conception of disinhibition reproduces Augustine suspicions of the temptations of the flesh, Cartesian dualisms that pitch mind against body, and Freudian struggles between the dark and dangerous instincts of the id and the controls of the conscience and civilised society, to produce the body essentially as a seat of volatile and violent drives, base instincts and dangerous passions.[14] Similar distinctions also structure Strudwick's wide-eyed depiction of gay BDSM activities. The school-boy terminology used to describe one such scenario is particularly revealing: 'What begins as standard slap 'n' tickle [swerves] beyond the agreed limits into punching, the pain of which is anaesthetised by the drugs' (2016).

Popular and scientific discourses of drug disinhibition also pepper most of the accounts of drug use in *Chemsex* (Fairman & Gogarty 2015), which spends a great deal of time fixating on 'slamming'. Though a majority of gay men who use chems refrain from this practice and administer their drugs in other ways (Hickson et al. 2016), the film is keen to deliver its hit and trades on mass fascination with this way of puncturing bodily boundaries and medical norms. *Chemsex* does include some footage of the many other ways in which chemsex practitioners administer drugs, and even contains rare footage of some care practices that gay men have devised to reduce harm in these settings: one fellow organising a group sex party at his home is shown going to the trouble of drawing up a detailed timetable to schedule his guests' G consumption as a way of ensuring their safety. There are also numerous accounts of what participants enjoy about sex on drugs and the intense pleasure they have experienced during chemsex sessions, but the bonds and transformations associated with these intensities are not explored in any depth or extensive detail unless they adhere to the consensual narrative of pain, destruction, tragedy and 'just desserts' (Young 1973). The film's over-determining narrative structure drains these scenes of any of their alternative pedagogical potential by training the viewer to lump all these practices together as the same monolithic, downward-spiralling, abject, sinister, inevitably treacherous phenomenon – a mission it accomplishes with the help of David Marle's persistent, jarring, brilliantly overwhelming soundtrack.

Changing the problem

Recent attempts to make chemsex public are so committed to normative intimacy that the many pleasures and possibilities associated with gay sex and drug use are only ever allowed to emerge as dangerous. This entertains their publics by giving them a bit of a gothic thrill, only to confirm them in their normality by delivering the requisite narrative of 'just desserts' and enrolling them in the consensual morality of liberal concern. In rendering what must, for many recipients, be unfamiliar and strange *legible* in familiar terms, this discourse confirms the law-abiding morality of the modular citizen. But for those whose sexual or consumption practices occasionally or more frequently deviate from juridical norms, this discourse only serves to amplify the dangers of illicit sex and drugs by dismissing the very possibility of agency in this cluster of practices. This produces chemsex as a fixed, intractable problem, in a dangerous and frightening pedagogy of exemplary negativity, which demonstrates not only that normative morality needs its monsters, but how – through sheer determination and unambiguous intentionality (discursive attributes projected onto the subjects of this discourse to define and isolate them) – public morality makes monsters out of sexually active gay drug users. To re-enact a quote from *Chemsex* – this time with novel feeling – 'I'm scared of this kind of perversion of the gay scene: It's pathological. There's something scary happening' (Fairman & Gogarty 2015).

Recent scientific and popular discourses of chemsex constitute it as a *case* in the medical sense: a pedagogical instance of exemplary negativity, a sign of personal pathology and communal disorder; an historic abnormality that teaches its publics something about the dangers of excessive sex and consumption. In this chapter, I have sought to counter this process by generating a critical perspective on what these ways of making chemsex public are producing. By fixating on the harms, dangers and most normatively disturbing instances of sex and drugs, these discourses dismiss and promote ignorance about whatever else is happening in this space that might open up more promising possibilities.

How might our approach to chemsex change if this conglomerate of practices were grasped otherwise, as an active scene of problematisation, its participants engaged in collective processes of experimentation, for example? By experimenting with different forms of enjoyment, new sensations and modes of feeling, and ways of encountering and being with other men erotically, chemsex participants might just be seeking new ways of feeling past injuries and/or experiencing present relations that transform their corporeal being in a manner that is not only intimate but intensely felt and highly material for them.[15] From this perspective, chemsex might consist of multiple, budding forms of lateral agency and possibilities for relationality; a collection of experiments that certainly have their risks and dangers, but nonetheless appear to hold some sort of promise for their participants.

Promise of what? Of transforming certain bodily capacities by generating new ways of feeling about oneself, one's world, one's life and one's sexual partners, perhaps: by re-enacting and re-working certain confronting or troubling scenarios (through BDSM activities, for example), some participants might be seeking to transform persistent apprehensions about being physical, vulnerable and intimate with other men (including strangers whose masculinity is threatening and/or exciting to them). Others may be seeking to convert residual anxieties into excitement and pleasure so that they can move on from certain things, or experience new sensations that make their bodies and their world feel different, or just enjoy themselves occasionally, like social drinkers who find sex easier or more enjoyable when drunk.

What then would happen if, like the practical ethic of HIV social research I discussed in Chapter 1, sexual health and drug service providers actually took the risk of constituting their clients/subjects/target communities as agents? Instead of confirming them in their normative identity by positioning them as hopeless, damaged, disordered victims, they might be constituted alternatively as members of shifting communities and networks, actively engaged in collective experiments to transform certain aspects of their situation and bodily being. What if public health experts prepared themselves to be surprised by the unexpected agency of those they seek to govern? How would this change the problem that confronts us? What if sexual health practitioners sought to learn *with* digital sexual subjects *from their* individual and collective experiments? The next chapter explores some preliminary possibilities.

Notes

1 Though largely resisted by community-based HIV agencies in Australia, such tendencies are evident at numerous discursive sites: the growing popularity of the concept of addiction as a way of explaining not only substance use, but also non-normative sexual activities and the use of digital media (Weiss 2005; Keane 2004; Cover 2016); a growing addiction-recovery movement that pits sobriety and normalcy against the sexual deviance and imputed depravity associated with the use of illicit drugs and hookup devices (Weiss 2005; Fawcett 2015); epidemiological discourses and public health practices that promote simplistic associations between substance use and HIV risk; and discourses of marriage equality that promote the latter in terms of its supposed benefits for HIV prevention.

2 The discourse of addiction has become available within consumer culture to problematise individual attachments to almost any sort of object, commodity or practice (Sedgwick 1993). For critiques of the application of the concept to the use of digital media see Cover (2016), and in relation to sexual activity, see Keane (2004).

3 An extensive literature on how queer sex play can reconfigure past, traumatic experiences of sexual violence exists. Most of this literature, which is ably summarised and discussed by Cvetkovich (2003), emanates from the work and thought of lesbian, gay, transgender and queer practitioners of S/M sex. My use of the term 'novel conceptual feeling' references the philosophy of A. N. Whitehead, for whom both the continuity of the subject and the determining nature of experience depend on re-enactment and repetition. Whitehead uses the term 'conformation' to describe situations in which 'simple physical feelings' are re-enacted and repeated, and 'causal efficacy' to describe the degree of continuity with which these re-enactments hold the subject in place as the same sort of subject and/or determine future experience. This process can be modified through what Whitehead calls 'subjective valuation' (which 'is the work of novel conceptual feeling'), which acquires importance and value through 'complex processes of integration and reintegration' and 'modifies the whole range of feeling in that concrescence' (Whitehead & Sherburne 1981, p. 57). In other words, while a given entity/being cannot entirely erase or remove past experiences (or 'simply physical feelings'), what can be modified is how an entity *feels* that 'simple physical feeling' through the process of its re-enactment. This operation alters the degree to which the past determines the present experience of that being/entity (its causal efficacy), *as well as* the nature of the subject/entity that eventuates through this process of 'subjective valuation' and 'novel conceptual feeling', which 'modifies the whole range of feeling' through the very process of re-enactment. Whitehead is not known for his work on erotic experience, sexuality or queer pleasure (he was a mathematician and philosopher whose work is most familiar among Christian theologicians!). Nevertheless, I find his work tremendously useful for conceiving bodily experience and experimentation, because he resists the modernist bifurcation of nature from culture, cognition from affect and matter from meaning (as can be seen in his expansive use of terms such as *feeling* and *prehension*). He further insists that the manner in which an entity *feels* the world affects what that entity is/becomes – a process that Foucault termed subjectivation (Foucault 1990). But these points are surely obvious to anyone who has found themselves sexed as a deviant subject and has had to learn to experiment with their situation – whether through thinking, reading, bodily play, sex, drug use or any other form of queer praxis, including dancing. Just after

AIDS deaths peaked in many Western urban gay centres, a dance track emerged to become a hit on queer dance floors around the world. The chorus repeated the claim, 'Music is the answer to your problems, keep on moving and you can solve them' continually over the entire 14 minutes of the original extended mix (Tenaglia 1998). Considered a revelation in its simplicity, the track resonated among its fans precisely because it enacts the challenge of 'solving problems' as a continuous process involving ongoing bodily movement, collective improvisation and experimentation in the presence of a repeated, endlessly extended beat that is variously felt and differently enacted by participants in dance events over the entire course of the record.

4 The availability and analysis of such data are highly variable in different health-care settings and public health jurisdictions, while the terms in which one understands the relation between substance use and sexual risk-taking (whether causal or a mere correlation), and how these terms come to matter, are frequently over-determined by official public health priorities. In London, such data became available when sexual health service-providers began including questions relating to drug use during sexual encounters on sexual history pro forma questionnaires collected from patients presenting for post-exposure prophylaxis. This data helped raise chemsex as a concern worthy of public health funding in the UK, even though many community-based agencies had long been aware of the multiple problems associated with use of methamphetamine and GHB/GBL among gay men and men who have sex with men (Stuart, D. 2017).

5 As Paasonen discusses, after the dotcom crash of the turn of the millennium, extensive efforts were made by digital tech companies to achieve greater resonance between technology corporations and their users, and these transformations are generally referred to as the Web 2.0 environment. This context saw the emergence of social software, more distributed forms of production and consumption (including 'prosumption'), and forms of functionality that streamlined and automated practices such as 'sharing' and uploading user content (2011, pp. 64–7).

6 'Set and setting' is a phrase taken from the work of psychiatrist Norman Zinberg (1986) that has been extremely influential in the fields of addiction research and drug and alcohol studies. Zinberg drew on extensive published data and case studies to develop an explanation for the fact that individual relations to drug use undergo significant changes according to their mindset ('set'), the type of drug used, the method of ingestion and the sociomaterial setting in which the drug is consumed ('setting'). Zinberg's work is recognised for offering a persuasive and influential explanation of why the same drug can affect different people in different ways, and indeed the same person differently in different times and places.

7 For a more extensive elaboration of this conceptual frame, which we designed to account for the activity of objects and devices in the transformation of everyday practices, see Hawkins et al. (2015, pp. 82–5).

8 Of course, enjoyment of this sociotechnical infrastructure is predicated on certain forms of privilege. The sexual culture built up around the use of these devices in urban centres depends in part on at least one of a given session participants' ability to access private accommodation in these locations – something that depends on economic affluence and/or cultural capital in the contemporary metropolis to an unprecedented degree. Members without such means sometimes use the apps to locate more than just sex in urban centres: for example, to find somewhere to sleep or just go and hang out, for company or to have a meal, to score free drugs, have a shower or get whatever else they can. Obviously, all sorts of opportunities

are made possible by these social networking devices, including transactional sex and drug dealing, usually by small-time dealers who are participants in this sexual culture themselves and sell their goods to known friends and less-known sexual partners (Thanki & Frederick 2016).

9 For example, John Frow writes, 'the *semiotic medium* and *physical setting* constitute a material and technical matrix within which genres are embedded. *They are not themselves a component of genre*, but they form part of the framing conditions which govern and may signal generic structure, and they have direct consequences for the structural organisation of genre' (2006, p. 73). But having 'direct consequences for the structural organisation of genre' is not quite the same thing as actively participating in the constitution of forms, practices and modes of engagement, the sort of agency with which I am investing these media here.

10 See above, note 4.

11 See Young (1973), whose analysis of the treatment of the drug user by mass media remains one of the best accounts of the sensationalising affects of mass media I know. Young breaks these affects down into a series of interconnected, mutually amplifying affective vectors that include excitement, intrigue, investment, disgust and moral indignation.

12 This was the name of a pamphlet produced by gay community activist Richard Berkowitz in consultation with Dr Joseph Sonnabend (Berkowitz 1983) which is generally recognised as one of the first instances of gay, sex-positive community self-education on potential methods of preventing the transmission of AIDS, and stands as one of the first formulations of 'safe sex' (Crimp 1987).

13 In a large opportunistic sample of gay men living in England assembled in 2014 (n = 15,360), Hickson and colleagues (2016) found that 8.3 per cent, 16.5 per cent and 12.5 per cent had ever used crystal meth, mephedrone and GHB/GBL respectively, while only 2.0 per cent, 5.3 per cent and 3.2 per cent had used each drug within the past four weeks, with 1.8 per cent of men reporting having injected any of these drugs in the previous twelve months. A higher prevalence of drug use has been found in London, but this is still much smaller than *Chemsex* (2015) would seem to suggest, with 11.1 per cent of London gay men reporting having used crystal methamphetamine in the previous twelve months (Melendez-Torres et al. 2016).

14 For an extended critique of how disinhibition operates in the discursive construction of crystal methamphetamine use, see Race (2009, pp. 174–9, pp. 149–55).

15 See my discussion of eternal recurrence, S/M sex and 'novel conceptual feeling' above, note 3.

References

Ahmed, A., Weatherburn, P., Reid, D. et al. 2016. Social norms related to combining drugs and sex ('chemsex') among gay men in South London. *International Journal of Drug Policy*, 38, pp. 29–35.

Ahmed, S. 2006. *Queer Phenomenology*. Durham: Duke University Press.

Arreola, S., Neilands, T., Pollack, L. et al. 2008. Childhood sexual experiences and adult health sequelae among gay and bisexual men: Defining childhood sexual abuse. *Journal of Sex Research*, 45, pp. 246–252.

Bech, H. 1997. *When Men Meet: Homosexuality and Modernity*. Chicago: University of Chicago Press.

Becker, H. 1963. *Outsiders*. New York: Free Press of Glencoe.

Berkowitz, R. 1983. *How to Have Sex in an Epidemic*. New York: News from the Front Publications. Retrieved from https://richardberkowitz.com/2010/06/29/blurbs-for-how-to-have-sex-in-an-epidemic/ [13 February 2017].

Berlant, L. & Warner, M. 1998. Sex in public. *Critical Inquiry*, 24(2), pp. 547–566.

Carnes, N. 2016. Gay men and men who have sex with men: Intersectionality and syndemics. In E. Wright & N. Carnes (eds.) *Understanding the HIV/AIDS Epidemic in the United States*. Dordrecht: Springer International Publishing, pp. 43–69.

Caron, D. 2014. *The Nearness of Others: Searching for Tact and Contact in the Age of HIV*. Minneapolis: University of Minnesota Press.

Cover, R. 2016. *Digital Identities*. Los Angeles: Elsevier.

Crimp, D. 1987. How to have promiscuity in an epidemic. *October*, 43, pp. 237–271.

Crowley, M. 1969. *The Boys in the Band*. London: Secker & Warburg.

Cvetkovich, A. 2003. *An Archive of Feelings*. Durham: Duke University Press.

Daskalopoulou, M., Rodger, A., Phillips, A. et al. 2014. Recreational drug use, polydrug use, and sexual behaviour in HIV-diagnosed men who have sex with men in the UK: Results from the cross-sectional ASTRA study. *The Lancet HIV*, 1(1), pp. e22–31.

Degenhardt, L., Roxburgh, A., Black, E. & Bruno, R. 2008. The epidemiology of methamphetamine use and harm in Australia. *Drug and Alcohol Review*, 27(3), pp. 243–252.

Delany, S. 1999. *Times Square Red, Times Square Blue*. New York: New York University Press.

Fairman, W. & Gogarty, M. 2015. *Chemsex*. London: Vice Productions.

Fawcett, D. 2015. *Lust, Men and Meth: A Gay Man's Guide to Sex and Recovery*. Wilton Manors, FL: Healing Path Press.

Ford, C. H. & Tyler, P. 1933. *The Young and Evil*. Paris: Obelisk Press.

Foucault, M. 1990. *The Use of Pleasure*. Trans. R. Hurley. New York: Vintage Books.

Foucault, M. 1997. Sex, power and the politics of identity. In P. Rabinow (ed.) *Ethics: Subjectivity and Truth*. London: Penguin, pp. 163–174.

Friedkin, W. 1980. *Cruising*. New York: CiP-Europaische Treuhand AG & Lorimar.

Frow, J. 2006. *Genre*. Oxon: Routledge.

Gogarty, W. & Fairman, M. 2015. *Chemsex*. London: Vice Media.

Green, A. & Halkitis, P. 2006. Crystal methamphetamine and sexual sociality in an urban gay subculture: An elective affinity. *Culture, Health & Sexuality*, 8(4), pp. 317–333.

Halkitis, P., Parsons, J. & Stirratt, M. 2001. A double epidemic: Crystal methamphetamine drug use in relation to HIV transmission. *Journal of Homosexuality*, 41(2), pp. 17–35.

Hart, T., Rotondi, N., Adam, B. et al. 2014. Use of party and play drugs mediates the association between childhood sexual abuse and unprotected anal intercourse with casual partners. *Canadian Journal of Infectious Diseases and Medical Microbiology*, 25(Supplement A), p. 94A.

Hawkins, G., Potter, E. & Race, K. 2015. *Plastic Water: The Social and Material Life of Bottled Water*. Cambridge: MIT Press.

Heredia, C. 12 February 2006. The same sex scene. *San Francisco Chronicle* [online]. Retrieved from http://www.sfgate.com/health/article/THE-SAME-SEX-SCENE-A-Serosorting-Story-Dating-2504382.php [31 January 2017].

Hickson, F., Reid, D., Hammond, G. & Weatherburn, P. 2016. *State of Play: Findings from the England Gay Men's Sex Survey 2014*. London: Sigma Research.

Hodges, M. 1980. *Flash Gordon*. Hollywood: Universal Pictures.

Hollinghurst, A. 2005. *The Line of Beauty*. London: Picador.

Hull, P., Mao, L., Kolstee, J. et al. 2016. *Gay Community Periodic Survey: Sydney 2016*. Sydney: Centre for Social Research in Health.

Keane, H. 2004. Disorders of desire: Addiction and problems of intimacy. *Journal of Medical Humanities*, 25(3), pp. 189–204.

King, M. 31 October 2015. Five ways to reclaim your sex life after booze, meth and other substances. *Queerty* [online]. Retrieved from https://www.queerty.com/five-ways-to-reclaim-your-sex-life-after-booze-meth-and-other-substances-20151031 [27 February 2017].

Kirby, T. & Thornber-Dunwell, M. 2013a. High-risk drug practices tighten grip on London gay scene. *The Lancet*, 381(9861), pp. 101–102.

Kirby, T. & Thornber-Dunwell, M. 2013b. New HIV diagnoses in London's gay men continue to soar. *The Lancet*, 382(9889), p. 295.

Latour, B. 2005. *Reassembling the Social*. Oxford: Oxford University Press.

Latour, B. & Weibel, P. 2005. *Making Things Public: Atmospheres of Democracy*. Cambridge: MIT Press.

Light, B. 2016. Creating sexual cultures and pseudonymous publics with digital networks. In R. Lind (ed.) *Race and Gender in Electronic Media*. Oxon: Routledge, Ch. 14.

Light, B., Fletcher, G., & Adam, A. 2008. Gay men, Gaydar and the commodification of difference. *Information Technology & People*, 21(3), pp. 300–314.

Mamo, L. & Fishman, J. 2001. Potency in all the right places: Viagra as a technology of the gendered body. *Body & Society*, 7(4), pp. 13–35.

McKirnan, D., Ostrow, D. & Hope, B. 1996. Sex, drugs and escape: A psychological model of HIV-risk sexual behaviours. *AIDS Care*, 8(6), pp. 655–670.

Melendez-Torres, G., Bonell, C., Hickson, F. et al. 2016. Predictors of crystal methamphetamine use in a community-based sample of UK men who have sex with men. *International Journal of Drug Policy*, 36, pp. 43–46.

Nietzsche, F. 2001. *The Gay Science*. Cambridge: Cambridge University Press (Orig. 1882).

Paasonen, S. 2011. *Carnal Resonance: Affect and Online Pornography*. London: MIT Press.

Parsons, J., Severino, J., Grov, C. et al. 2007. Internet use among gay and bisexual men with compulsive sexual behavior. *Sexual Addiction & Compulsivity*, 14(3), pp. 239–256.

Parsons, J., Grov, C. & Golub, S. 2012. Sexual compulsivity, co-occurring psychosocial health problems, and HIV risk among gay and bisexual men: Further evidence of a syndemic. *American Journal of Public Health*, 102, pp. 156–162.

Quinn, B., Stoové, M., Papanastasiou, C. & Dietze, P. 2013. An exploration of self-perceived non-problematic use as a barrier to professional support for methamphetamine users. *International Journal of Drug Policy*, 24(6), pp. 619–623.

Race, K. 2009. *Pleasure Consuming Medicine*. Durham: Duke University Press.

Race, K., Lea, T., Murphy, D. & Pienaar, K. 2016. The future of drugs: Recreational drug use and sexual health among gay and other men who have sex with men. *Sexual Health*, 14(1), pp. 42–50.

Raj, S. 2011. Grindring bodies: Racial and affective economies of online queer desire. *Critical Race & Whiteness Studies*, 7(2), pp. 1–12.

Sedgwick, E. K. 1993. Epidemics of the will. In E. K. Sedgwick (ed.) *Tendencies*. Durham: Duke University Press, pp. 130–142.

Shakespeare W. 2015. *Macbeth*. London: Penguin (Orig. 1623).

Stall, R., Friedman, M. & Catania, J. 2008. Interacting epidemics and gay men's health: A theory of syndemic production among urban gay men. In R. Wolitski, R. Stall & R. Valdiserri (eds.) *Unequal Opportunity: Health Disparities Affecting Gay and Bisexual Men in the United States, 1*. New York: Oxford University Press, pp. 251–274.

Strudwick, P. 2016. This is what chemsex is doing to gay men: Inside the dark, dangerous world of chemsex. *Buzzfeed News* [online]. Retrieved from https://www.buzzfeed.com/patrickstrudwick/inside-the-dark-dangerous-world-of-chemsex?utm_term=.rbMJKWEze#.dcxmqAJ54 [9 February 2017].

Stuart, D. 2013. Sexualised drug use by MSM: Background, current status and response. *HIV Nursing*, 13, pp. 1–5.

Stuart, D. 2016. Chemsex is a complicated public health issue. *Indetectables* [online]. Retrieved from http://indetectables.es/david-stuart-chemsex-is-a-complicated-public-health-issue [10 February 2017].

Stuart, D. 2017. *Funding chemsex in the UK*. Personal communication with D. Stuart on 12 February, Sydney.

Tenaglia, D. 1998. Music is the answer. *Tourism* (LP record). United States: Twisted American Records.

Thanki, D. & Frederick, B., 2016. Social media and drug markets. In *Internet and Drug Markets*. Publications Office of the European Union, Luxembourg, pp. 115–123.

Tinkcom, M., 2011. 'You've got to get on to get off': *Shortbus* and the circuits of the erotic. *South Atlantic Quarterly*, 110(3), pp. 693–713.

Weiss, R. 2005. *Cruise Control: Understanding Sex Addiction in Gay Men*. Los Angeles: Alyson Books.

Whitehead, A. N. & Sherburne, D. 1981. *A Key to Whitehead's Process and Reality*. Chicago: University of Chicago Press.

Woo, J. 2013. *Meet Grindr: How One App Changed the Way We Connect*. Seattle, WA: Amazon Digital Services.

Woolgar, S. 1991. Configuring the user: The case of usability trials. In J. Law (ed.) *A Sociology of Monsters*. London: Routledge, pp. 58–99.

Young, J. 1973. The myth of the drug taker in the mass media. In S. Cohen & J. Young (eds.) *The Manufacture of News*. London: Constable, pp. 314–322.

Zinberg, N. 1986. *Drug, Set and Setting: The Basis for Controlled Intoxicant Use*. New Haven: Yale University Press.

8 Speculative intimacies

Some less acknowledged possibilities of smartphone use

As we saw in Chapter 7, online hookup devices play a central role in chemsex discourse. It is surprising, then, that there has not been more attention within it to how gay men actually use them. Instead, online hookup devices tend to be prematurely stabilised as objects that enable rapid sexual turnover, make drugs more accessible and divorce sex from other social contexts to produce social isolation. Each of these claims no doubt captures certain realities, but smartphone apps have other affordances, and there are other ways of engaging with them and enacting 'the problem'.

Beyond the issue of chemsex, online hookup devices have been subject to extensive criticism in gay popular culture, the terms of which nonetheless echo certain aspects of their problematisation within chemsex discourse. As a Sydney gay man put it in a widely shared blog post,

> the community has been decimated by the Internet . . . gays everywhere have become a sick group of animals who have completely lost their ability to interact on any authentic level. . . .We are an un-community. We have become a consumer product. We are the iGays.
>
> (endracismandhomophobia 2012)

In this posting and in others like it, the Internet is said to have destroyed the authenticity of sexual community by divesting gay men of their social capacities and turning them into commodities. Key elements of this critique also appear in the pages of queer theory. For example, Tim Dean contrasts a romanticised yesteryear of street and cinema-based cruising with the 'degraded form that cruising for bareback sex often takes, namely, hooking up online' (2009, p. 176), in a searching discussion that pits 'public and social' sex against 'sex in front of a computer monitor, which tends to be solitary' (p. 186), and is said to embody 'a purely instrumental approach to the other' (p. 194) and participate in a 'troubling privatization of intimacy' (p. 177). These analyses pit a romanticised past of more 'authentic' forms of sociability against an apparently decimated, technologically saturated present. And yet they wrestle with a question of undeniable significance: what forms of relationality are the sex venues of the present eliciting?

One of the formative ideas of modern social and political theory is that the rise of the technical object can be held responsible for the demise of community. In this habit of thought, industrial objects (whether technologies, objects or commodities) are said to have demolished any prospect of collective identity or authentic community, extracting people from their communal relations by creating dangerous fixations that only serve to alienate them (Race 2009, pp. 71–9). But the authentic community that constitutes the nostalgic object of mainstream critique is beset with paradoxes in the gay context, and becomes somewhat perverted in the process (not such a bad thing). The sexual communities of urban gay culture are not the familiar zones of homogenous identity and transparent recognition lamented within mainstream critique after all, but have always been animated by practices of 'stranger sociability' – a feature that many queer theorists not only underline but tend to go to town on (Berlant & Warner 1998; Delany 1999; Warner 2002; Dean 2009).

Is there then another way of casting the problem that pays more attention to how technical objects mediate sociability? One approach would be to make use of the conceptual tools from economic sociology I drew on in Chapter 6. Economic sociology may seem like an odd place to go to look for creative ways of conceiving of gay sexual culture, but the frequent reference to the 'sexual marketplace' within digital sex discourse is suggestive, and the pragmatist approach adopted within this work has certain benefits. For Michel Callon, a market transaction is a special type of encounter that differs from other forms of social relation (such as those of gift and obligation) in specific ways: '*Once the transaction has been concluded the agents are quits:* they extract themselves from anonymity momentarily, slipping back into it immediately afterwards' (1998, p. 3, author's emphasis). On Callon's argument, this feature of market transactions is not intrinsic or self-evident but must be specifically assembled: 'It is not easy to make this relationship of strangeness compatible with the unavoidable fact that the agents are in touch with each other during the transaction' (1998, p. 3). Significantly, this involves a certain amount of technical labour, not only on the part of human subjects but also that of material objects and settings. To enable a market transaction, *framing devices* are needed to disentangle the agents in question from other networks and relations. But these framing devices are often incommensurable with one another or ineffective. Any encounter thus framed as a market transaction may become subject to 'overflowing' (1998, p. 18).

This pragmatist approach to market arrangements directs attention to how certain material settings and devices frame certain encounters as 'no-strings' or commitment-free, while conceiving of how such frames may fail to contain the relations they arrange (what Callon terms overflowing). This may give us a better grasp on the forms of connection and estrangement that have characterised gay sexual sociability – its specific textures and qualities, its varieties of intimacy and disconnection, the sorts of attachments that arise in any given relation. Callon's approach lends itself to a more nuanced perspective on the qualitative nature of such relations; the degrees of reciprocity, care, indebtedness, commitment, neglect or disregard that may emerge from different sexual occasions. At the same time, it refuses to confer on any one way of framing these encounters some essentialised status – 'one is not born a commodity, one becomes it', as he quips (1998, p. 19). This refusal becomes particularly significant when considering the unlikely emergence of 'sexual community' in modern urban gay centres.

Online hookup devices tend to frame the sex they enable as 'no-strings' or commitment-free, and on this basis they can be understood as framing devices. But they are certainly not without precedent in gay culture: indeed, framing devices have long been significant in the formation of gay relations and urban sexual communities. A number of well-known studies of early twentieth-century homosexual life discuss how parks, streets and washrooms afforded a degree of privacy 'that could only be had in public' (Chauncey 1996, p. 224; see also Humphreys 1970; Bech 1997; Delany 1999). Chauncey (1996) gives a nuanced account of the multi-varied use of washrooms for sex between men in twentieth-century Manhattan. While many of the men who used these spaces for sexual liaisons were poor and had little access to other kinds of private space, the apparent lack of emotional involvement characteristic of sex in these spaces also made these venues attractive to different groups of men who, for various different reasons, wished to 'isolate [these encounters] from the rest of their lives and their identities' (1996, p. 252). It is easy to see how these environments served as framing devices, enabling men to compartmentalise and frame their sexual encounters. Part of their appeal lay in the access they provided to a critical mass of men seeking sexual contact; but it also consisted in the anonymity these venues afforded for a range of different users and the means they offered for severing any ongoing personal involvement.

Such means were later carried over into the purpose-built architectures of modern gay life such as the sauna and sex-club, which have served as meeting points and social venues but also spaces of convenience. These structures enabled participants to disentangle themselves easily from further engagement should they so desire. Modelled on architectural prototypes such as the arcade and shopping centre (Chisholm 2005), they aimed to promote consumer attachments while making these same attachments available to debt-free exchange and limited personal involvement (McFall 2009). From backrooms to web-camming facilities, we can begin to appreciate how the topic of framing devices includes a wide array of objects. For example, the enduringly popular 'glory hole' serves quite literally as a framing device, providing circumscribed access of mouth to penis (or penis to mouth or other body parts) in a way that brackets other features of the participants or their connection. Some may see this contraption as the height of dehumanised and impersonal sex. But what it also makes available is an occasion of mutual enjoyment and affective intensity among otherwise unlikely intimates or sexual partners.

In suggesting market devices have long played a constitutive role in gay sexual cultures and communities, I hope it is clear my purpose is not to critique these communities – indeed, the architectures of romance are no less contrived. Rather, I want to push back a little against the assumption that the digital moment uniquely commodifies gay sexual practice, and suggest instead that gay communities have long navigated the work of such framing devices. Indeed, it could be argued that the rich and complex fabric of twentieth-century sexual communities has depended on techniques for circumscribing the erotic and social relations that make it up to enable a variety of distributed, more modulated intimacies and bonds to flourish. Fleeting sexual acquaintances may evolve over time and get reconfigured in different contexts to take their place within extended friendship networks or just become available to mutual recognition and constitute a sense of ordinary belonging (Warner 2000; Adam 2006). This point interested Michel Foucault, who described the 'multiple intensities, variable colors, imperceptible movements and changing forms' of homosexual relations, proposing:

> homosexuality is a historic occasion to reopen affective and relational virtualities, not so much through the intrinsic qualities of the homosexual but because the 'slantwise' position of the latter, as it were, the diagonal lines he can lay out in the social fabric that allow these virtualities to come to light.
>
> (1997, pp. 137–8)

My suggestion in this chapter is that digital sex arrangements simply offer new ways of assembling such diagonal lines. As Gibson (1977) taught us, the affordances of an object depend on the predispositions and goals of the creature encountering it, but this does not exhaust what may be done with the object; such encounters are also subject to creativity. Hence the speculative or open-ended character of the ensuing analysis: the realisation of possibilities is not determined in any empirical sense, but anticipates (indeed requires) co-invention.

'Looking to play?'

Chemsex or PnP can therefore be grasped as a marginal set of activities emerging from a more general attitude to sex and its social function that has long circulated within gay culture, namely the framing of sex as *play*. Play is a key term that motivates and sustains much of the sex arranged between men online. 'Looking to play?' is one of the most common questions employed to initiate conversation via this medium. The question does a number of things: first, it attempts to establish whether the recipient of the message is aiming to arrange an offline sexual encounter, indicating a key rationale and ostensible motivation for online participation in general. Second, it characterises that encounter as casual, fun and obligation-free. Third, it indicates the possibility of a number of other modes of online participation – from checking messages, to 'having a look', to random chat, to casual browsing – that may be differentiated from actually looking to play. 'Looking to play' is the online equivalent of cruising, but it differs from cruising in significant ways – most obviously in *how* it takes place and its reference to the visuality of the digital interface. Chemsex or PnP is a subset of this more general framing of sex. Not all of the sexual play arranged online is PnP, to be sure, because it most often does not involve the use of drugs. But PnP would not take the forms it does in the absence of this precedent.

The frequent deployment of the term play affords further insight into the social possibilities of the sexual encounters arranged within hookup culture. In *The Sociology of Sociability*, Georg Simmel and Everett Hughes (1949) situate the play-form as a constructive component of social formation. Simmel and Hughes conceive of play as a non-instrumental form of association in which the exchange of stimuli is the governing principle and in which personality, serious content and substantive ends are suspended or displaced to cultivate the pleasures of association. Indeed, the authors deem the need or desire of an individual for serious results or instrumental ends to interrupt the play-form. Describing sex as play dislodges sex from narratives that prioritise the mutual development of biographical intimacy, clearing a space for sex in the assembly of affective associations that Simmel and Hughes term sociability. For these sociologists, play has an important social and associative function and this is why they make the paradoxical observation that 'men can complain both justly and unjustly of the superficiality of social intercourse' (p. 261). Tellingly, the charge of superficiality has long been levied at gay sexual culture, but usually with none of the sociological promise with which Simmel and Hughes invest it here.

This perspective on play as an associative activity also resonates with Bruno Latour's proposal to replace conventional approaches to sociology with 'associology'. In *Reassembling the Social* (2005), Latour rejects the tendency, common within the social sciences, to frame 'community' or 'the social' as explanatory devices with their own laws and properties that transcend specific instantiation (2005, pp. 9–12). Instead, he promotes the project of tracing how heterogenous elements become *associated* in different forms or assemblages over time (hence the term 'associology'). Latour's approach has particular value for social and cultural studies of HIV. The importance of community is widely cited in gay men's health promotion but it tends to be reified as an ideal or stable form that is defiled by subsequent transformations. By adopting an 'associological' approach, in which play is located as a key mechanism of association, we can track some of the ways in which sexual community is currently being assembled while paying careful attention to the performative impacts of objects, technologies and devices in this process.

Smartphone affordances

Online hookup devices provide cruising with a digital and textual materiality that differs from the conditions characterising some of the longer-standing venues of casual sex. As we have seen, this enables various forms of controlled disclosure prior to any sexual encounter – e.g. sexual interests or HIV status – and these capacities have been implicated in the emergence of new modes of partner sorting and risk prevention. Unlike some of their Internet predecessors, gay hookup apps have generally not prompted HIV disclosure until relatively recently, leaving such disclosure to take place through the mechanism of private messaging which constitutes the primary terrain in which sexual arrangements are made. Various forms of screening and negotiation take place in this terrain, in which users gradually release information to indicate what they are interested in and set parameters around what might take place. This often involves treading a fine line between protecting one's identity and self-exposure and entails various forms of sexual and vernacular literacy. Many differently situated participants appreciate this affordance. For example, Aaron, a transman I interviewed, explained to me how useful it has been for him to have a discussion about practices, desires and possibilities in the safety of relative anonymity prior to agreeing to meet up with a prospective partner.

In previous research, I have analysed instances of chat from my own participation in online hookup culture, which I have captured using the screen-cap function on my smartphone and reproduced (Race 2015). I used these bits of digital communication to discuss the operation of various forms of 'veiled disclosure' during online chat (Figure 8.1). Veiled disclosure allows online cruisers to 'test the waters' with thinly veiled signals about themselves or their sexual interests that are assumed to be legible to those in the know but less decipherable to unsympathetic parties. It is often used to communicate stigmatised interests or attributes, such as being HIV-positive, wanting to have sex without condoms, wanting to have sex on drugs or simply to protect one's identity and anonymity.

There are two main points to make about this strategy. The first is that it mediates the terms of access that members have to each other, and on this basis ought to temper the anxiety about unprecedented accessibility associated with online hookup devices in representations such as *Chemsex* (Fairman & Gogarty 2015). To make an obvious point, one is not obliged to participate in whatever activities might be proposed or 'introduced' to them online. Users actively make use of personal chat to sort for partners and arrange activities they feel comfortable with. It becomes possible, for example, to organise a group sex session in which participants are more aware of what they are entering into by setting parameters or disclosing information around participants' HIV status, drug use or other risks associated with the arrangement. In short, while online hookup devices enable new forms of sexual access, the communication of risk and safety via these mechanisms mediates the sexual encounters that eventuate. The second point to emphasise is that this capacity relies on developing vernacular, digital literacies around sex, drugs and HIV prevention possibilities. Online chat is not random in its signification but is organised according to genre – that is, the cultural conventions that organise

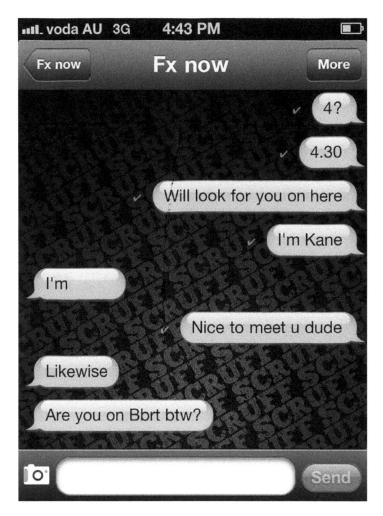

Figure 8.1 Veiled disclosure.

Scruff conversation, author's own

participants' expectations of the exchange and the meanings they make of it. This is evident, for example, in the screen-capped exchange taken from my own use of Scruff in Figure 8.2, in which the fellow I am chatting with responds to my 'naïve', research-oriented question 'what if I said I was neg?' with the amusing retort 'U would have by now lol'. This exchange demonstrates how such conversations are bound by vernacular conventions that in turn become available for reflexive comment, vernacular learning, reflection, adaptation and improvisation. These conventions tend to be specific to a given cultural location: cultivating the relevant literacies would equip participants

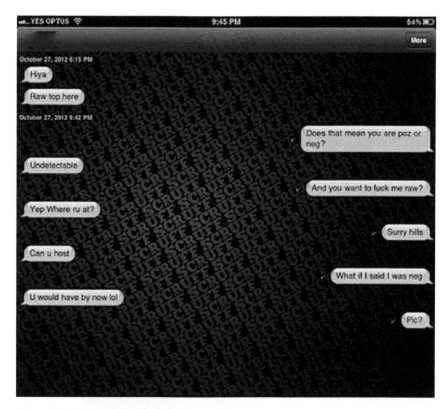

Figure 8.2 Conventions of disclosure.
Scruff conversation, author's own

to recognise and deal with the (often) veiled forms of disclosure and invitation that surround stigmatised activities.

While it would be nice to claim my use of smartphone functions to collect this 'data' as some original innovation in research methods, I admit I adapted this research device by borrowing from what was already a common practice in gay popular culture.[1] Capturing and storing digital images and chat conversations has emerged as a gay cultural practice in its own right, and now operates as a means of collecting and sharing erotic information and memorabilia within gay friendship circles and sexual networks. Such records serve various personal and social functions: a source of recollection, fantasy, information-exchange, gossip, boasting, comparison, evidence, vernacular learning, archiving, betrayal, exposure, speculation and ammunition. That is to say, these bits of digital data can be seen as an example of how digital devices are creating new forms of sexual sociability; they are bound up in the constitution of new intimacies, social relations and forms of collective learning.

This affordance acquires particular significance in relation to questions of HIV prevention. For example, in jurisdictions where HIV non-disclosure is criminalised, HIV-positive individuals have been known to screen-cap chat in which they have disclosed their status in case they are called upon to furnish evidence. In HIV-related Facebook discussion groups such as *PREP Facts* (Jacobs 2015), members regularly share screen-capped images of their personal chat exchanges to open them up for collective commentary, analysis and problematisation. The trajectory of this data from private to public implicitly runs the risk of breaching ethical sensitivities, but when principles such as de-identification are followed, they can be seen to generate new, collective, practical and ethical capacities. These sharing practices are often undertaken in the interests of what I have called 'counterpublic health' (Race 2009) and can be understood to generate collective contexts in which 'intimate relations and the sexual body can . . . be understood as projects for transformation among strangers' (Warner 2002, p. 122).

Erotic speculation and the eventuation of sex

'There is no textbook for how to be a safe gay man in modern times, in a changing healthcare world, in a changing app world, in a changing hooking up technology world', David Stuart remarks when interviewed in the documentary *Chemsex* (Fairman & Gogarty 2015). He has a point, though there is some question in my mind about whether the didactic pedagogy evoked by the figure of the textbook sufficiently grasps the interactive, emergent and co-constructed nature of the pleasures, risks and relational and speculative possibilities of digital sex. Digital chat constitutes a new textual and material space in which sexual activities and desires are not simply stated but co-constructed in conversational format, either as a prelude to or irrespective of a sexual encounter. Some participants describe the latter mode of erotic speculation as 'random chat'. This genre is significant, if only because such a space of erotic exchange among relative strangers has never existed in precisely this format before. Erotic chat serves as a means by which people select and screen for sexually compatible partners, as I discussed above. But these exchanges can also constitute a form of play themselves, insofar as they hover in a precarious space that teeters between pure exchange and the pursuit of instrumental ends (i.e. actually hooking up). This ambiguity and prevarication about intentions is experienced by many as a source of frustration, as becomes evident in the frequent appearance on people's profiles of statements such as 'not into hours of endless chat', etc. But for some participants, these interactions constitute an erotic activity in and of themselves, in which various pleasures and desires are proffered in digital text, sometimes supplemented by selfies and explicit self-pics which are sent to solicit appreciation from the other party and indicate sexual intentions or desired scenarios. These conversations may extend to previous sexual experiences, or sexual desires and fantasies more broadly, or familiar scenes from porn films, etc. As well as learning about certain possibilities and stating personal parameters, erotic speculation enables participants to experiment with ideas about what they might want, constituting a space in which fantasies materialise into more concrete opportunities, intentions and desires – or else remain in the realm of chat and fantasy.

Co-constructed fantasy may shape expectations of offline encounters, either structuring these encounters or leading to disappointment, insofar as the ensuing encounter fails to live up to the pre-constructed fantasy of it. Adam and colleagues have considered the sense in which 'the crystallization of their fantasies in the texts that constitute the vehicle for their interaction is akin to the joint construction of a script' (Adam et al. 2011, p. 507). They offer some evidence that talking positively about unprotected sex online prior to meeting a given partner correlates with unprotected sex in practice, even when condom use is stated as the initial intention. Particularly interesting here is the suggestion that sexual desires, intentions and even identities do not precede the online encounter in any simple sense, but can be understood to emerge from it through a process of eventuation. This tells us something about the generative properties of this sexual infrastructure. Since online hookup devices are not simply a space of representation but also a vehicle for interaction – the material mechanism for arranging sexual encounters – they produce new proximities between chat, pornography and real-time sexual encounters that may generate new amalgamations of fantasy and practice. Many cruising websites feature prominent links to other sites that enable the streaming of pornographic films, including the increasingly popular genre of barebacking pornography.[2] Here, viewing pornography may be interspersed with practices of sexual searching in practical constellations that produce new relays between pornographic scenes, the material arrangement of sex and what actually plays out in these encounters.

My point here is not to entertain a simplistic model of media effects but rather the opposite; to signal the significance of attending to the relations that constitute a sexual occasion and its material possibilities, whether good or bad. This point was brought home to me in an interview with an articulate HIV-negative Sydney gay man with over three decades' experience of casual sex with younger men (generally in their twenties), whom he has met primarily through online hookup devices since they have been available:

> The whole Internet thing and the whole, you know, camming and porn industry – because it's so everywhere, you know, like because it's so accessible – people, especially young guys, seem to think that it's all, everything's very disposable and it's like, 'Well I,' you know, like their imaginations are fired up with all these visuals that they watch all the time and it's almost like, when they meet a guy they want just to recreate what really turns them on from what they've seen, and they want it *here*, and they want it *now*. And it doesn't really work like that. Because you need to meet a person. You need to interact with that person.

You need to then . . . you need to just calm down, you know, rather than put the horse, the cart before the horse. And this is what I find a lot of guys are doing: they're putting the cart before the horse when it comes to what their fantasies are rather than just allowing things to eventuate and unfold.

(Jason, fifty years old, HIV-negative)

The point of citing this discussion is not to denigrate 'young people these days', but to differentiate between different modes of sexual pedagogy and consider the different orientations to the sexual encounter they embody. Though certainly not averse to porn consumption himself, Jason draws a distinction between two different approaches to the sexual encounter. In his experience, partners who are most directly tutored in the scripts of online porn tend to approach the sexual encounter with a predefined script they seem determined to enact. He contrasts this with a different approach that takes the time to allow some dynamic between the participants to 'eventuate and unfold'. This relational dynamic, informed by embodied experience, seems to me to be very close to the sort of responsive attentiveness I have been advocating in previous chapters, where what is most significant is how various (human and nonhuman) elements come together to constitute an event in all its contingency.

Responsive attentiveness involves paying attention to the way in which various forces, relations, affects and objects converge to *make something available* or *allow something to emerge*. Paul Rabinow and Bruno Latour each convey relevant perspectives in the following passages:

[F]rom time to time, and always in time, new forms emerge that catalyze previously existing actors, things, temporalities, or spatialities into a new mode of existence, a new assemblage, one that makes things work in a different manner and produces and instantiates new capacities. A form/event makes many other things more or less suddenly conceivable.

(Rabinow 2002, p. 180)

We collectively elaborate an emerging and historical event which was not planned by any participant and which is not explainable by what happened before the event or what happens elsewhere. All depends on the local and practical interactions in which we are presently engaging.

(Latour 1994, p. 50)

The pleasures and risks of digitally arranged sex also eventuate relationally and sometimes overflow their initial framing. Acknowledging these pleasures and risks involves an art of paying attention.

The Ancient Greeks used the figure of the pharmakon (which can be translated as drug) to refer to the instability of objects and identities, and their potential to function as both poison and cure depending on the circumstances they enter into. Isabelle Stengers uses this figure to convey the need for a certain training of the attention that brings into play 'connections between what we are in the habit of keeping separate' (2015, p. 62). As she puts it, 'the instability of the pharmakon has been used again and again to condemn it . . . [but this] allows the question of the appropriate attention, the learning of doses and the manner of preparation, to be done away with' (Stengers 2015, p. 100). These remarks are applicable to any of the elements and identities that come together in digital sex encounters, but they take on particular salience when attending to chemsex arrangements.

PnP sessions

This returns us to the riskier scene that has come to be known as chemsex, or PnP, or 'wired play', which I have come to think of as the attempted construction of a pornographic elsewhere (or heterotopia) insofar as it is regarded as an exceptional or extraordinary scene of erotic intensity. This is where the use of drugs comes in (though not necessarily for all participants). Hurley and Prestage (2009) characterise such practices as 'intensive sex partying': I am making a case for further attention to the objects and devices that come together in the construction of such occasions: parties cannot be understood apart from the material devices and infrastructures that constitute them as specific occasions. They do not take place in abstract space; rather, the space of the party is enacted through specific practices, objects, devices and arrangements.

A preference for chemsex or PnP may be stated on one's profile or proposed during chat, where it indicates the desire to engage in sexual play for quite a while, often with more than one partner or a sequence of partners over several hours or even days. While the focus of these occasions is ostensibly sex, such arrangements may actually comprise a number of activities, including chilling, chatting, watching porn, browsing profiles and a range of other group and individual activities. Crystal methamphetamine is used in this setting to effectuate certain capacities: it enhances sexual sensation, but also keeps users awake and alert, enabling them to maintain the sort of focus and fixation required for browsing online profiles and watching porn for extended periods. Crystal use may also delay ejaculation (sometimes indefinitely), which suggests that 'getting off' is not necessarily the prioritised aim of the sexual encounter. Rather, what becomes valued is the capacity to maintain focus on various sexual activities and possibilities, and the stamina or staying power required to sustain these erotic engagements.

Crystal functions as a baseline drug for these purposes, and is usually smoked through a glass pipe or sometimes injected. The drug Gamma-Hydroxybutyrate (GHB) is sometimes used to initiate or reinitiate sexual activities, such that an extended session typically goes through various phases – sex, chilling, chatting, smoking, taking G, sex – that correspond or alternate with the high that GHB produces (which can last about an hour).

Crystal may also be smoked alone, prior to any sexual encounter, to get into a sexual frame of mind, dispense with everyday inhibitions, browse profiles, initiate sexual conversations, formulate fantasies and build up the courage and confidence to follow through on these. If these attempts do not amount to anything (and often they do not), the result can be disappointment, loneliness and frustration, affects that may be intensified by the highs and lows of the drug. The promise of instant sexual availability may clash with the sense of non-delivery that is actually a common experience of online sexual searching, and this may compound residual feelings of despair and isolation.

PnP can be considered a specific instantiation of a more general mode of experimentality or play that characterises participation in these scenes more generally. What is being experimented with here? Often it is masculinity, and the question of what men can do with each other, bodily and relationally, to erotic effect (McInnes et al. 2009). This is carried out through actual sexual contact, but also through random chat, shared viewing and discussion of porn, exchanging stories about other encounters, 'camming' with remote erotic spectators, and sharing information about previous experiences or images of previous sexual partners. In Deleuze's Spinozist ethology, variations in intensity always correspond with some variation in extensive relations, and it would seem chemsex practitioners are keen to experiment with these intuitive possibilities (Deleuze 1992). However much enjoyment is experienced in a given configuration of participants, bodies, relations, texts and devices, there will often come a time when people disentangle themselves from the situation and begin to browse online profiles on their devices in a bid to find further participants. This may give rise to further erotic speculation: banter and gossip about particular profiles, previous experiences or sexual encounters, and the issuing of invitations to new participants. Or it may turn what was previously a scene of sexual exhilaration into something that resembles nothing so much as a tense but dull scene of office administration, with each participant locked to their computers and devices, obsessively searching for newcomers to join the session. In any case, what we have here is a suspension or extenuation of enjoyment: a will to novelty but also intensive differentiation. While some sorting for partners generally takes place, this is manifestly not the atomised or isolated activity that some critics suppose – a fact that becomes evident in the frequent reference to 'buddies looking', 'hanging with mates' and 'group sessions', as well as practices of collective viewing and searching. Together, these activities embody a will to sexual sociability that manifests as the motivational logic of this sexual assemblage. This characteristic is illustrated in this profile shot cropped with permission from an informant's Manhunt profile in 2011 (Figure 8.3), which depicts the member and his buddies browsing online profiles in a *mise en abyme* that substitutes entirely here for the more conventional individual portrait. As this instance suggests, different configurations of collective activity are a distinctive feature of this constellation of practices, and may be regarded as a logic that energises and sustains group play sessions.

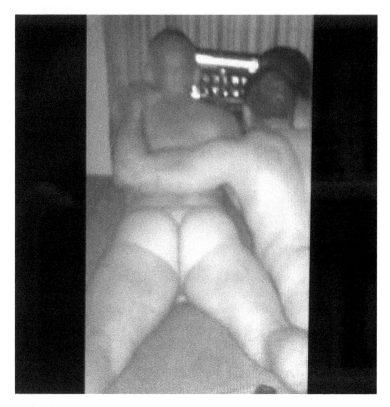

Figure 8.3 Hanging with mates.

Image cropped with permission from the Manhunt profile of anonymous interview participant

There is of course significant potential for a range of accidents to occur during PnP sessions. But we should not discount the capacity of participants to manage such risks and reduce the harms associated with the relevant forms of drug use.[3] With regard to HIV transmission, I have already indicated that digital chat mechanisms can be used effectively to disclose risks and have conversations about HIV status and the possibilities of infection. Moreover, with the shift to biomedical prevention, new chemical infrastructures are now in play in different locations that mediate the risk of sex without condoms in material ways. Even in the context of 'drug-fuelled' multi-partner sex without condoms (as 'chemsex' is often sensationally characterised), the risk of HIV infection is reduced if the viral load of HIV-positive participants is suppressed by the use of antiretroviral therapy, and/or when HIV-negative participants are using pre-exposure prophylaxis (PrEP). With increased rates of HIV test-ing, early initiation of antiretroviral therapy on the part of HIV-positive individuals, uptake of PrEP by at-risk individuals and effective adherence, the risk of HIV infection can be reduced (though the transmission of other STIs will not necessarily be mitigated). Taken together, these developments oblige us to confront what some may consider an equally scandalous but nonetheless recognisable possibility: the prospect of 'drug-fuelled HIV prevention'.

Meanwhile, though risks such as addiction and dependence are commonly framed as intrinsic properties of drugs such as crystal, *whether* and *how* such risks eventuate varies according to the practices and contexts in which these drugs are used, which calls for further consideration of their 'set and setting' (Zinberg 1986).[4] If gay dance culture was popularly perceived to involve the dispersion of sexual energies to the more diffuse eroticism and communal affection of the dance floor, the use of digital hookup devices typically locates gay sexual socialising at home and frames sex as the primary modus operandi of such encounters. The stigmatised status of crystal methamphetamine can lead to practices of self-isolation:

> With crystal, particularly, it doesn't really matter what I'm doing, I just get really focused on it. [Laughs] So, so if I'm on Scruff [a gay geo-locative app] or, and there would generally be porn in the background as well, like I'd generally be watching porn and being on Scruff at the same time, [At home? Or. . .] At home, yeah, yeah. And, I s'pose there's a bit of shame for me around using crystal so I don't really wanna use it with other people. Again which is why I tend to spend a lot of time chatting before I actually hook up.
>
> (Dan, thirty-two years old, HIV-negative)

The storage and use of these drugs in the home of the user, and the fact that methamphetamine is not self-limiting like ecstasy, make habitual use and increased dependence a real possibility: the drug can be integrated relatively easily into everyday personal, domestic and labour routines. For some users, the pleasures and intensities of online hookups come to punctuate what are experienced as increasingly confined and desperate terms of everyday life, leading to increasing use and dangerous self-isolation. Other users learn ways of managing their crystal use over the long term that do not interfere with their everyday responsibilities, while still others just get bored with this attachment and substitute it with others, like dog-walking, cooking, drinking, knitting, gambling, other social activities or friendships. Various attempts have been made in the critical literature to reformulate addiction in terms that avoid the pathologisation of the user or the demonisation of illicit substances (Sedgwick 1993; Keane 2002). If gay recovery advocates promote complete abstention from erotic speculation and zealous compliance with normative intimacy (King 2015), critically informed experts suspend a priori judgement about what constitutes a dangerous attachment and indeed what constitutes intimacy: alcoholism is said to involve a 'narrowing of the drinking repertoire', for example. In this sense it is not much different to normative intimacy and exclusive coupledom (Keane 2004). Who knows what dangers or problems such attachments may pose in specific situations? We all need attachments: the question of whether an attachment is good or bad is a matter for subjective valuation (Latour 1994). From my perspective, addiction can be understood as a fixation or repeated attachment that begins to obliterate the subject (or their capacity to persist in the world) before it can be dislodged or destabilised. If overcoming addiction involves destabilising or reconfiguring a fixed attachment, then experimental and speculative activities may well play a role in dislodging those that are deemed to pose certain dangers and substituting them with others, contra the pious absolutism of some recovery proponents.

As Zinberg (1986) argued, the 'set and setting' of drug use mediate its dangers and effects in proven ways. On this point, it is necessary to emphasise that the governmental assault on queer nightlife and party spaces discussed in Chapter 2 exacerbates the dangers associated with drug use by driving it underground or behind locked doors. As I have already suggested, the sequestering of methamphetamine consumption to private, domestic settings lends itself to heavier use and growing dependence. When it comes to G consumption, if accidents or emergencies do occur, participants are often too scared of the legal, moral and personal repercussions of being implicated in such illicit disapproved activities to seek assistance from the relevant authorities or service-providers. But alternatives are possible. In their early work on practices of harm reduction at gay dance events in Sydney, Southgate and Hopwood (2001) identified the existence of lay experts ('network nannies') who enact various harm reduction practices within their friendship circles and teach initiates how to do so. In Chapter 2, I discussed the formation of the Rovers, a group of volunteers who rove around gay dance events on the lookout for people in trouble, especially in the context of GHB-related emergencies (Gonçalves et al. 2016). Over the course of undertaking research and activism in this area, I have been approached by a number of people who report often taking on a role they describe as the 'G nurse' or 'party nurse' during group chemsex sessions. Not only are these men keen to learn more about how they could enact this role better; they are speculating about the possibility of using smartphone apps for home oxygen saturation and vital sign monitoring during GHB incidents to help determine when it is safe to let someone sleep and when to call emergency services, and have initiated conversations with clinicians with a view to developing guidelines about such possibilities. The organic emergence of the party nurse as a recognised figure within chemsex circles not only presents new opportunities for peer-based education and care, it also paints a very different picture of the sorts of relations and possibilities that animate home-based partying than we have so far encountered. With better resourcing and less dogmatic moral policing, LGBT community health agencies could better articulate their harm reduction programmes with emergent, relatively hidden subcultural figures and practices such as the party nurse, who already serve to enhance the safety of these spaces and events for many participants.

Conclusion

In this chapter I have sought to describe some of the distinctive features, activities and modalities of sex arranged between men online. I have argued that these activities can best be understood as a form of play and erotic speculation in which men experiment with bodily possibilities so as to produce more expansive experiences of pleasure and masculinity. I have argued that sexual media can be approached as a specific structure of entanglement that gives rise to new capacities, interactions and affordances. This allows people to sort for preventive identities and desires, to co-construct fantasies derived from various erotic sources and to arrange multiple forms of sexual encounter. That is to say, this sexual infrastructure is generating new modes of material participation in gay sexual culture, new forms of community and a range of speculative intimacies. Gay men's health promotion might seek to engage some of the emergent genres of sexual/risk negotiation I have begun to describe here, with the aim of equipping participants with more attentive ways of navigating them.

Another aim of this chapter has been to experiment with practices of acknowledgement: to find a register for grasping practices that are typically disavowed, making them available for more expansive consideration. As a form of play, online hookups exist somewhere on a continuum between playful exchange and instrumental ends, which means they may not resolve into the private couple form easily or readily. Indeed, even those who claim to be searching for 'a reason to delete this profile' (i.e. a boyfriend) typically express interest in 'some fun along the way'. Noteworthy here is the potential disconnect between people's normative identifications and their actual sexual practices. At a time when marriage and monogamy increasingly monopolise the public discourse of gay relations, the capacity to maintain a loose web of sexual friendships is perhaps more available, more accessible and more widely accessed than ever before. But these sociomaterial arrangements are rarely acknowledged or given institutional support; instead they emerge as tacit possibilities that the new infrastructures of digital sex make available. The mechanism of the buddy list, a feature that allows participants to keep track of their favourite members, lends itself readily to the arrangement of repeat encounters. Online devices and apps thus present the possibility of arranging sexual encounters in real time that are relatively casual and spontaneous but also recurring, such that they might involve known acquaintances, or relative strangers, or some combination; depending on who is online, who is looking, who is nearby and who makes themselves available. This is an historically distinctive way of arranging erotic and intimate life that has social and communal potential. These devices and practices are participating in the construction of a specific sphere of sociability and amiable acquaintance among men in urban centres that prioritises sex as a catalyst for connection and sociability. While online hookups are frequently framed as 'no-strings' or commitment-free, they are always subject to various forms of overflowing

(Callon 1998), in that they may generate affective bonds and identifications that change the texture of what Michael Warner has termed 'stranger sociability' in urban gay centres (Warner 2002). By paying attention to the pleasures, risks, activities and encounters that are variously emerging from and animating this space, we are better able to grasp them and engage the social assemblages they are generating.

Notes

1 This is not the first time that personal information systems have informed sexuality research, of course. The Stud File kept by the gay professor Samuel Steward is an early example of how elements of (what were once) new information systems found their way into expert forums. Steward recorded details of his every sexual encounter on individual cards in a card catalogue system which served as an archive as well as a means of arranging repeat encounters. His meticulous maintenance of this file made him one of A. F. Kinsey's most significant informants (Spring 2010).

2 See Dean (2009, pp. 97–144) for the most comprehensive discussion of bareback porn to date, and Paasonen (2011) for an excellent analysis of the affective dynamics of online pornography among different viewers.

3 While common wisdom positions sexual risk-taking as a bio-psychological consequence of intoxication, the correlation between chemsex and HIV infection is much more complex and contingent on a range of other factors and variables. The sexual networks of men who use drugs for gay sex are characterised by a higher prevalence of HIV-positive participants and lower rates of condom use, often as a result of attempted serosorting (Rawstorne et al. 2007). Lower rates of condom use within this sexual milieu may affect the prevention practices of HIV-negative participants, who may wish to conform to the sexual and social norms they perceive to be operating in these spaces. Meanwhile, the 'extended sessions' facilitated by methamphetamine can involve a higher number of sexual partners and a greater likelihood of anal and other physical abrasions that increase susceptibility to HIV and BBV infection. In general, HIV-negative men who participate in these sexual networks are likely to have a higher number of HIV-positive sexual partners (Rawstorne et al. 2007). Meanwhile, the higher prevalence of injecting drug use within these sexual networks increases the risk of exposure to blood-borne viruses such as hepatitis C, which may occur through sharing drug and/or sex equipment and/or through specific sexual activities (Hopwood et al. 2015). Precautionary measures that may be effective in other contexts become more precarious in these conditions, putting those who participate in networks of sexualised drug use at greater risk of HIV, BBV and ST infection.

4 'Set and setting' is a phrase taken from the work of psychiatrist Norman Zinberg (1986) that has been extremely influential in the fields of addiction research and drug and alcohol studies. Zinberg drew on extensive published data and case studies to develop an explanation for the fact that individual relations to drug use undergo significant changes according to their mindset ('set'), the type of drug used, the method of ingestion and the sociomaterial setting in which the drug is consumed ('setting'). Zinberg's work is recognised for offering a persuasive and influential explanation of why the same drug can affect different people in different ways, and indeed the same person differently in different times and places.

References

Adam, B. 2006. Relationship innovation in gay male couples. *Sexualities*, 9(1), pp. 5–26.

Adam, P., Murphy, D., & De Wit, J. 2011. When do online fantasies become reality? The contribution of erotic chatting via the internet to sexual risk-taking in gay and other men who have sex with men. *Health Education Research*, 26(3), pp. 506–515.

Bech, H. 1997. *When Men Meet: Homosexuality and Modernity*. Chicago: University of Chicago Press.

Berlant, L. & Warner, M. 1998. Sex in public. *Critical Inquiry*, 24(2), pp. 547–566.

Callon, M. 1998. *The Laws of the Markets*. Oxford: Blackwell.

Chauncey, G. 1996. Privacy could only be had in public: Gay uses of the streets. In J. Sanders (ed.) *Stud: Architectures of Masculinity*. Princeton: Princeton Architectural Press, pp. 244–267.

Chisholm, D. 2005. *Queer Constellations*. Minneapolis: University of Minnesota Press.

Dean, T. 2009. *Unlimited Intimacy*. Chicago: University of Chicago Press.

Delany, S. 1999. *Times Square Red, Times Square Blue*. New York: NYU Press.

Deleuze, G. 1992. Ethology: Spinoza and us. In J. Crary & S. Kwinter (eds), *Incorporations*. New York: Zone Books, pp. 625–633.

Endracismandhomophobia. 2012. The iGays are way too sick [weblog]. Retrieved from https://stopracismandhomophobiaongrindr.wordpress.com/2012/07/20/the-igays-are-way-too-sick-turn-off-the-life-support/ [24 February 2017].

Fairman, W. & Gogarty, M. 2015. *Chemsex* [film]. London: Vice Media.

Foucault, M. 1997. Friendship as a way of life. In P. Rabinow (ed.) *Ethics: Subjectivity and Truth*. London: Penguin, pp. 135–140.

Gibson, J. 1977. The theory of affordances. In R. Shaw & J. Bransford (eds.) *Perceiving, Acting, and Knowing*. New York: Wiley, pp. 127–143.

Gonçalves, D., Kolstee, J., Ryan, D. & Race, K. 2016. Harm reduction in process: The ACON Rovers, GHB, and the art of paying attention. *Contemporary Drug Problems*, 43(4), pp. 314–330.

Hopwood, M., Lea, T. & Aggleton, P. 2015. Drug, sex and sociality: Factors associated with the recent sharing of injecting equipment among gay and bisexual men in Australia. *International Journal of Drug Policy*, 26(2), pp. 210–213.

Humphreys, L. 1970. *Tearoom Trade: Impersonal Sex in Public Places*. London: Aldine.

Hurley, M. & Prestage, G. 2009. Intensive sex partying among Sydney gay men. *Culture, Health & Sexuality*, 11(6), pp. 597–610.

Jacobs, D. 2015. *PrEP Facts* [online discussion group]. Retrieved from https://www.facebook.com/groups/PrEPFacts/ [27 February 2017].

Keane, H. 2002. *What's Wrong with Addiction?* Melbourne: Melbourne University Press.

Keane, H. 2004. Disorders of desire: Addiction and problems of intimacy. *Journal of Medical Humanities*, 25(3), pp. 189–204.

King, M. 31 October 2015. Five ways to reclaim your sex life after booze, meth and other substances. *Queerty* [online]. Retrieved from https://www.queerty.com/five-ways-to-reclaim-your-sex-life-after-booze-methand-other-substances-20151031 [27 February 2017].

Latour, B. 1994. On technical mediation: Philosophy, sociology, genealogy. *Common Knowledge*, 3(2), pp. 29–64.

Latour, B. 2005. *Reassembling the Social*. Oxford: Oxford University Press.

McFall, L. 2009. Devices and desires: How useful is the 'new' new economic sociology for understanding market attachment? *Sociology Compass*, 3(2), pp. 267–282.

McInnes, D., Bardley, J. & Prestage, G. 2009. The discourse of gay men's group sex: The importance of masculinity. *Culture, Health & Sexuality*, 11(6), pp. 641–654.

Paasonen, S. 2011. *Carnal Resonance*. Cambridge, MA: MIT Press.

Rabinow, P. 2002. *French DNA: Trouble in Purgatory*. Chicago: University of Chicago Press.

Race, K. 2009. *Pleasure Consuming Medicine*. Durham: Duke University Press.

Race, K. 2015. 'Party and play': Online hook-up devices and the emergence of PnP practices among gay men. *Sexualities*, 18(3), pp. 253–275.

Rawstorne, P., Digiusto, E., Worth, H., & Zablotska, I. 2007. Associations between crystal methamphetamine use and potentially unsafe sexual activity among gay men in Australia. *Archives of Sexual Behavior*, 36(5), pp. 646–654.

Sedgwick, E. K. 1993. Epidemics of the will. In E. K. Sedgwick (ed.) *Tendencies*. Durham: Duke University Press, pp. 130–142.

Simmel, G. & Hughes, E. 1949. The sociology of sociability. *American Journal of Sociology*, 55(3), pp. 254–261.

Southgate, E. & Hopwood, M. 2001. The role of folk pharmacology and lay experts in harm reduction: Sydney gay drug using networks. *International Journal of Drug Policy*, 12(4), pp. 321–335.

Spring, J. 2010. *Secret Historian: The Life and Times of Samuel Steward, Professor, Tattoo Artist, and Sexual Renegade*. New York: Farrar, Straus & Giroux.

Stengers, I. 2015. *In Catastrophic Times: Resisting the Coming Barbarism*. London: Open Humanities Press.

Warner, M. 2000. *The Trouble with Normal*. Cambridge, MA: Harvard University Press.

Warner, M. 2002. *Publics and Counterpublics*. New York: Zone Books.

Zinberg, N. 1986. *Drug, Set and Setting: The Basis for Controlled Intoxicant Use*. New Haven: Yale University Press.

9   Conclusion

The queer chemistry of counterpublic health in digital times

Queer counterpublics have been seen as a significant resource for gay men's HIV prevention and harm reduction (Berlant & Warner 1998; Warner 2002; Race 2009). This chapter works with this concept (which I will elaborate further shortly) to think about how critical collectivities of sex might operate in the digital context. The question is particularly timely right now, since we are in the middle of a radical transformation in sexual geography in many Western contexts, and digital technologies are no doubt implicated in whatever will emerge from this. In my home town of Sydney, regarded by many as the historical and symbolic centre of Australian gay life, the intensity of the state assault on 'nightlife' in the last couple of years has left many of us reeling, as one by one bars, clubs, parties and the experience of street-life that connects them seem to be vanishing through closures, curfews and intensive policing. As I discussed in Chapter 2, the urban conditions that once made it possible to imagine Sydney's LGBTIQ population as a heterogenous but inclusive sexual community are changing rapidly and inexorably.

While some see these changes as a welcome by-product of the increasing acceptance of gays and lesbians into mainstream life, the governmental erasure of urban sexual scenes has occurred alongside a proliferation of homonormative discourses that prioritise marriage equality and normalising conceptions of gay life. In their eagerness to present gays and lesbians as respectable, everyday folk, these discourses frequently assume sex, drug and HIV-phobic forms (Liu 2015, p. 2). Their capacity to shut down constructive responses to the realities of sex, drugs and HIV infection will not be lost on anyone who has followed online discussions of any of these topics recently. These remarkably polarised and polarising debates are conspicuous for their denigration of those expressions of queer or embodied life that are taken to compromise the public image of sexual minorities as normal upstanding citizens. Needless to say, such instances of 'in-group purification' (Goffman 1963, p. 108) further stigmatise practices that require more constructive, generous forms of attention and open acknowledgement, especially with respect to their public health implications.

My thinking emerges from a concern with how the changing topology of gay life bears the potential to undermine the possibilities of 'counterpublic health' (Race 2009). This term raises the significance of collective contexts of embodied reflexivity for those areas of public health characterised by a tension between public morality and the practical ethics of care devised by subordinate groups. HIV prevention and harm reduction are key examples of counterpublic health, since both require some acknowledgement of embodied practices (gay sex or drug use) that are difficult to acknowledge or have a sensible discussion about in the public sphere proper without these issues being sensationalised and assuming Gothic proportions. The stigmatised status of these activities means they are more likely to be addressed constructively in forums that maintain some critical distance from – or fly under the radar of – the norms and imperatives of the public sphere proper. This chapter revisits some of the most influential theorisations of queer counterpublics to recall their basic operating principles and think about how they might be realised in the digital context. No doubt, new opportunities for counterpublic activity will emerge as subjects conventionally identified as audiences and consumers of media become 'networked and mobilized', to adopt Mizuko Ito's characterisation of networked publics (2008, p. 2). But the exemplification of queer counterpublics in the critical literature has drawn so extensively on the cultural forms of late twentieth-century urban sexual subcultures in the West, pre-Internet, that it is worth trying to distil some of their key principles and consider how they might be taken forward and enacted given the increasing prominence of digital sex as a basic touchstone of gay sexual culture.

Sex in public

Digital sex is thinly but dismissively characterised in the critical literature that advances queer counterpublic theory. In their landmark essay 'Sex in Public', Berlant and Warner (1998) present digital sex as one of two rather meagre options remaining for those who want to access urban gay sexual culture following the devastating impact of Mayor Giuliani's zoning laws on New York's queer sexual culture. One option the authors flag is to cruise for sex in dangerous inaccessible areas on the waterfront; the other is to 'cathect the privatized virtual public of phone sex and the Internet' (1998, p. 192). In either case, 'the result will be a sense of isolation and diminished expectations for queer life, as well as an attenuated capacity for political community', the authors argue (p. 192). Given the essay's general critique of the privatisation of sex, I think we know how we are meant to feel about the Internet.

The association of digital sex with privatisation, conceived as a politically regressive and disabling tendency, is repeated in other influential analyses of changes in urban sex cultures. In Chapter 8 I discussed Tim Dean's (2009) depiction of online cruising as a solitary experience that involves a 'troubling privatization of intimacy' (p. 177) and embodies 'a purely instrumental approach to the other' (p. 194). Dean draws on Samuel Delany's *Times Square*

Red, Times Square Blue to contrast an ethic of *contact* to the practice of networking, and associates each of these respective practices with different modes of sexual encounter. If *contact* depicts a mode of sociality premised on the possibility of having the sort of unplanned 'erotic, interclass encounters' once associated with gay cruising in urban space (p. 188), networking is said to be 'class bound and membership oriented' (p. 191), and predicated on 'unprecedented control over one's erotic engagement with others' (p. 193).

I will return to these characterisations of the sexual encounter later in the chapter. For now, I want to situate these remarks within the broader theorisa-tion of queer counterpublics, with particular reference to the work of Michael Warner. Counterpublics are generally conceived in these pages as rhizomatic structures consisting of relays among various forms of media circulation and embodied inhabitations of sexual space. Warner defines a counterpublic as a multicontextual space for the circulation of discourse that 'maintains an awareness of its subordinate status' in relation to hegemonic discourse (2002, p. 119). Unlike community (a much more familiar term within the neoliberal governmentality of public health), counterpublics are said to come into being 'through an address to indefinite strangers' (p. 120). In this sense, they are 'oriented to stranger circulation in a way that is . . . constitutive of member-ship and its affects' (p. 122). Participation 'does not simply reflect identities formed elsewhere . . . it is one of the ways by which its members' identities and formed and transformed' (p. 121). In other words, the identities and subjectivities of counterpublics are *emergent*. The condition of stranger socia-bility means that participation in any public or counterpublic will necessarily involve encounters with alterity. Warner invests counterpublics with particu-lar significance for the critical transformation of gender and sexuality on this basis, suggesting 'a culture is developing in which intimate relations and the sexual body can in fact be understood as projects for transformation among strangers' (2002, p. 122).

Counterpublic health and 'risked estrangement'

Certainly, the examples Warner gives of social relations mediated by queer counterpublics are suggestive of the transformations associated with queer responses to HIV (Race 2009). The AIDS crisis sparked unprecedented experiments in 'forms of intimate association, vocabularies of affect, styles of embodiment, erotic practices, and relations of care and pedagogy', to recite Warner's terms (2002, p. 57). The affective capacities that enabled this popu-lation to respond so creatively and effectively to the public health emergency are difficult to dissociate from those that proliferated more generally within the urban assemblages that sexual minorities had fashioned for their enjoy-ment over the late twentieth century, with their particularly queer mix of sexual and social affordances. But since 'Sex in Public' depicts the vitality of counterpublics as especially vulnerable to changes in the government of urban space (Berlant & Warner 1998), it is easy to form the impression that accessible face-to-face environments are centrally implicated in their realisation. One would think there is little basis for characterising any one form of sexual media as *ipso facto* privatising. Such a determination would at least need to concern itself with the relays that occur between forms of media and the domains of everyday life in which 'gender and sexuality can be lived' (Warner 2002, p. 57). If counterpublics are multicontextual in their emergence and operation, they cannot be confined to any one particular genre of media. But in much queer critique, digital sex tends to feature as the province of isolated cultural dopes and instrumental consumers.

The queer enthusiasm for face-to-face environments could be attributed to the sense in which the infrastructures of urban gay life have traditionally been predicated on encounters with strangers, or at least facilitated such encounters. The loss of visible, accessible, face-to-face communal infrastructures might register more precisely therefore as the loss of contexts of stranger sociability that once effectuated 'the necessity of risked estrangement' – a condition that Warner situates as generative of counterpublic activity (2002, p. 122). Certainly, many have benefited from the opportunities gay sexual infrastructures have provided to engage erotically with strangers; opportunities that can be conceived as occasions to experiment with different ways of experiencing one's intimate exposure to others. Such occasions have allowed many queer people to gain an affective handle on apprehensions of hostility and estrangement that have been formative for them, allowing them to convert these apprehensions into sources of potential pleasure and enjoyment through erotic re-mediation. Since intimacy is conventionally associated with the private couple, the idea it might emerge from ongoing exposure to what random strangers make erotically available is particularly queer. The reduction of opportunities for collective exposure to the unknown bodies of others would certainly produce 'diminished expectations for queer life' from this perspective. When certain intermediating contexts that have traditionally afforded such opportunities are subject to eradication or are otherwise caused to change their form significantly, this loss can be keenly felt, as recent contests over the policing of nightlife in cities such as Sydney demonstrate (Race 2016). But while live sexual scenes provide one context for erotic exposure to strangers, they are not the only one conceivable, nor should they be seen as some essential precondition of queer counterpublic activity. I would argue that *exposure to alterity* might operate as the constitutive condition of the particular adventures in intimacy that queer counterpublics are said to make available. As Nietzsche put it, '"We" humans must remain strangers to ourselves, "out of necessity"' (cited in Ansell Pearson 1997, p. 15).

Queer events and sheer disclosure

Abstracting these principles form Warner's work offers a more precise sense of the losses entailed in the disappearance of certain institutions of gay life. One only need consider the significance of events like Mardi Gras for community responses to HIV in this country. In Gary Dunne's (1992) novel, *Shadows on the Dancefloor*, the Mardi Gras party emerges as a particularly significant scene, not only for processing the horrors of AIDS, but also for fostering intimate encounters among differently situated social actors. Drawing on my own experience of these events, we might include among this vernacular list of actors: nice boys and poz pigs; lesbians and drag queens; white-collar professionals and transgender sex workers; party boys and straights; junkies, politicians, opera queens, doctors, teachers, students, police (both uniformed and off-duty), firemen, janitors, clergymen and countless others. The culture of Mardi Gras may in this sense be conceived as a particularly dynamic and volatile scene of what danah boyd (2010) has termed 'context collapse', in which worlds and bodies, the public and the private, the social and the sexual unpredictably collide: in which you were just as likely to run into your high school French teacher; or a friend from primary school; or a work colleague in the arms of a trick you'd rather forget; or your long lost Uncle George in circumstances you thought were about getting trashed, or cruising for sex, or dancing vigorously on a podium in a state of undress, or finding a boyfriend. Naturally, this collision of different social worlds elicited considerable apprehension among participants. Sometimes it generated feelings of humiliation associated with unwanted exposure. But it also created new occasions for self-disclosure, communal pleasure, care, understanding and support; unlikely friendships and intimacies, playfulness, hilarity and gossip that kept the party going long after the lights went up in the pavilions. The encounters these events occasioned between differently situated individuals gave rise to new affective capacities and a diffuse but embodied sense of collective belonging. This enabled those affected by the crisis to craft new ways of withstanding its devastating impacts and confront its challenges, and find new ways of enjoying each other, despite the enormous losses sustained by many over this period.

My point is not to grumble and grizzle, 'we knew how to party when I was a lad'. I only want to illustrate the generative energy of what Warner terms *risked estrangement*. Clearly these spaces did not represent some realm of authentic, unmediated, communal experience. They were certainly mediated – by the music, the drugs, the lights, the dancing, the architecture of venues, the care services and the performativity of the dancefloor – a complex assemblage that produced 'different ways of imagining stranger sociability and its reflexivity' (Warner 2002, p. 121). They had their exclusions, to be sure, and no doubt some participants experienced these events as unpleasantly alienating at times. But at its best, this culture was guided by what Robert Payne has called 'a promiscuous methodology that prefers to see *what might happen* when disparate elements are allowed to come into a new intimate relation' (2015, p. 14). Warner pays similar attention to the transformative potential of queer encounters when he conceives queer counterpublics as a 'space of coming together that discloses itself in interaction' (2002, p. 122).

The safety of networking

My reference to dana boyd's work in this discussion of Mardi Gras suggests an analogy with networked publics, which are also said to be prone to
'context collapse' – the unanticipated blurring of public and private boundaries (boyd 2010). But while online hookup devices share certain features with
the social networking platforms that boyd conceives as networked publics,
they also differ in certain ways that bear outlining. A principal difference is
that online hookup devices prioritise point-to-point communication – dyadic
exchanges between members framed as private. On social networking sites
like Facebook, the Friendship list serves to circumscribe the possibilities of
contact and visible connection among members and demarcate shared spheres
of acquaintance. This is generally not the case with gay hookup devices. Users
rarely have access to any representation of other users' social or sexual networks,
though of course there are exceptions (MacKee 2016). Instead, members'
access to each other is mediated by a range of technical functions and modes
of engagement: screening, sorting, filtering, pre-selecting, winking, unlock-
ing, searching and blocking are common gestures. (Many of these gestures
might be considered to concretise or 'make durable' what psychologists have
termed 'anti-process' – the preemptive recognition and marginalisation of
undesired information by the interplay of mental defence mechanisms (Arndt
et al. 1997).) While apps targeting the gay market are blissfully free of the
complex algorithms found on mainstream dating sites that purport to determine compatibility and mediate access between members on this basis, much
of the appeal of these devices – gay and straight alike – is the promise they
extend to access members of interest and exclude others according to pre-
defined criteria, governed by the principle of what Miso Matsuda has called
'selective sociality' (2005). Together these functions furnish users with the
promise of control over the terms of their erotic engagement with others,
and are generally predicated on the idea that people know what they want in
advance from an intimate encounter.

  While digital technologies thus provide new opportunities for intimate
encounters between strangers, one can see how the controlled framing of
these encounters might be considered so pre-determining that it effectively
forestalls the development of peripheral relations in the vicinity of sex, such
as those that have characterised the development of urban sexual communities historically. To look for sexual partners today, the digital context asks
me to format my erotic curiosity according to a list of pre-defined interests
and preferences, which it presumes I have already established. I cannot help
but wonder, had I always organised my search for sexual partners this way,
whether I ever would have encountered the butch dykes or drag queens or
girly boys that turn out to have played such a significant role in my sexual
formation and sociopolitical outlook. What opportunities would there have
been to develop frank, affectionate bonds with queers from different walks
of life, had we not been thrown together on dance floors, bars and gutters

in collective states of disrepair? Sharing a sexual space with other people – including those you don't consider your 'sexual type' – can lead to mutually transformative exchanges that are not only surprising, but produce new ways of feeling, understanding, relating with others and being, not to mention much richer, wider, more playful distributions of intimacy.

Consider the sort of subject that online hookup devices format and configure. They anticipate a pre-calculative sexual subject who is presumed to know what they want in advance; whose preferences and interests are imagined to precede their worldly engagement with others. For all the benefits and convenience of restrictive search terms, these functions minimise the chances of having to engage with unlikely sexual and social others in the course of realising one's sexual interests. Not only does this militate against the development of the complex relational fabric constitutive of urban sexual communities: I do not think sexuality works that way. Public sex cultures can expose you to things you never imagined you wanted, even if in retrospect your desire for them can come to seem hardwired into your basic sense of yourself and your sexuality. The most exhilarating pleasures are often those you never imagined could function as a source of enjoyment; that *move* you beyond yourself and make new ways of experiencing yourself and relating to others possible. 'Styles of embodiment are learned and cultivated', Warner observes. They may be 'altered through exchanges that go beyond self-expression to the making of a collective scene of disclosure' (2002, p. 63). This is what it means to conceive of pleasure as an *event* (Foucault 2011, p. 389): an occasion that mediates and transforms the identities of all those who are party to it.

Loving encounters

In *In Praise of Love* (2012), Alain Badiou makes some scathing remarks about online dating that nevertheless might take this discussion in significant new directions. For Badiou, love is an opportunity to construct an ongoing relation through which 'you learn to experience the world on the basis of difference and not only in terms of identity' (2012, p. 16). Love is an adventure that springs from a chance encounter characterised by contingency, randomness, risk, surprise and unexpectedness. At its most interesting, love poses the question: 'what is the world like when it is experienced, developed, and lived from the point of view of difference and not identity?' (Badiou 2012, p. 22). Badiou gives such encounters 'the quasi-metaphysical status of an *event*, something that doesn't enter into the immediate order of things' (p. 28). Although he conceives of love as an entirely worldly affair, 'it is an event that can't be predicted or calculated in terms of the world's laws. Nothing enables one to pre-arrange the encounter' (p. 31).

This investment in the chance encounter informs Badiou's disparaging remarks about online dating: Badiou charges online dating with enacting 'a safety-first concept of "love". It is love comprehensively insured against all risks' (p. 6). By enabling you to screen and select your partner carefully, 'by searching online – by obtaining, of course, a photo, details of his or her tastes, date of birth, horoscope sign, etc.' (p. 6), and 'all those long, preparatory chats' (p. 31), the primary mode of social engagement within this medium is the 'risk-free' option of shoring up one's identity. The preemptive technologies of online dating work against the existential possibility love offers 'to construct a world from a decentred point of view other than that of my mere impulse to survive or re-affirm my own identity' (p. 25). When contingency, chance and surprise are managed out of the encounter, the creative possibilities of love are depleted.

Badiou's perspective on love cleaves closely to the long-term private couple as a privileged source of existential insight. Needless to say, it is informed by heteromasculinist presumptions that remain largely unexamined in his analysis. He differentiates love from friendship on the basis that 'friendship doesn't involve bodily contact or any resonances in pleasure of the body [!]' (p. 36). The philosopher is apparently oblivious to the joys of 'friends with benefits': it does not seem to occur to him that a wider distribution of love or sexual intimacy might generate more expansive perspectives on otherness. But at least Badiou has the decency to permit same-sex lovers' access to the perspective on difference that love is said to afford, and his account has the additional value of dislodging childbirth and monogamy from their pivotal status as consecrating measures of love's authenticity. Moreover, there are certain parallels between Badiou and Warner's thinking here, however surprising that might seem. Both authors emphasise 'risked estrangement' as a source of transformation within scenes of intimacy, and in both accounts it is the unpredictability of this exposure to others that imbues intimacy with its distinctive transformative potential. Badiou's conception of the intimate encounter as a dynamic event invokes a particular orientation to temporality, to open futures, that gives us a sharper appreciation of the temporality of self-transformation. Meanwhile, Warner supplies ways of extending the transformative energy of intimacy beyond the bounds of the private couple.

Logging back on

I want to return to digital culture now, armed with the spoils of these theoretical and personal excursions. None of these philosophers seem to like digital romance very much, but reading them alongside each other provides new ways of thinking about how intimacy re-meditates the self and may be re-mediated in turn. Badiou's reflections help to reformulate what queer critics have diagnosed as a troubling privatisation of intimacy in cultures of digital sex. With his bodily existence already well serviced by the public sphere as conventionally formulated, Badiou is less concerned with questions of privacy or publicness. Usefully, though, he diagnoses *aversion to risk* as the problem that online dating enacts: its reinforcement of identity, its preemptive shutting down of access to others and to difference. Badiou's critique has the advantage of reformulating the problems of digital intimacy by transposing them from a spatial to a temporal register. This allows us to imagine the eventuation of queer life in other ways. Queerness need not take the topographical form of a territory to be defended, but might instead denote a particular manner of relating to the world of others that affirms open-ness to alterity. This leaves us with a practical question in the digital context that is topological rather than topographic in nature: how can these adventures in intimacy be made more expansively and collectively accessible?

Online dating prioritises point-to-point communication, as I have mentioned: dyadic exchanges that are carefully framed to give the impression of relative privacy. But as danah boyd has argued (2010), the bits-based nature of digital environments introduces distinctive affordances to digital communication: persistence, replicability and scalability are particularly relevant for the present discussion. In Chapter 8 I considered how people use the screen-cap function to capture intimate exchanges for various purposes. Interactions that were once ephemeral can now be copied, stored and circulated. One potential scene of circulation is the networked public of social networking sites such as Facebook, Instagram and Twitter. It is now common for people to post instances of digital sex chat on these apps for various illustrative and demonstrative purposes, including on pages devoted to matters of concern such as HIV prevention.

This example indicates the relevance of cross-platform studies for counter-public activity in the digital context. Some trajectory from private to public is necessary to make digital intimacy 'go beyond self-expression to the making of a collective scene of disclosure' (Warner 2002, pp. 62–3). Digital media make personal interactions replicable and scalable in a manner that is more widely accessible than ever, while the multimodal nature of digital culture presents extensive opportunities for unanticipated exposure to indefinite others – some dangerous, others more promising or transformative. In this book I have proposed another way of conceiving this move from the private into wider sphere of sociality: 'frame-overflowing' (Chapter 8). What is needed are concrete analyses of the ways in which 'private' digital interactions are embedded and dis-embedded in other scenes of circulation.

Frame analysis provides further resources for counteracting the selective sociality prioritised by online hookup devices. It might even be used to query the self-consolidation that Badiou associates with the pre-screening tools of dating websites. Certainly, these tools can be used to curb contingency and all-too-narrowly frame the terms of one's engagement with others. But as Michel Callon has suggested (1998), frames are always subject to overflowing, and they can never completely contain the relations they act upon or control for the unexpected. For all their appeal to pre-calculative intentionality, moreover, no one could claim that digitally arranged intimate encounters are devoid of surprises (or at least, no one who is actually familiar with these sites or has spent some time using them). As an older girlfriend of mine who recently joined Blendr and Tinder told me excitedly, going online has opened up a world of erotic possibilities for her that she had all but given up on, but 'there's a lot to learn' and you have to 'manage your expectations':

'keep them low and expect the unexpected' is the policy she is working with but admitted, 'that's half the fun of it really'.

Other people adopt creative strategies to address the tendency of digital frames to produce such selection bias. One man I interviewed always arranges to meet guys in a bar after chatting on apps to get a sense of how things might unfold in practice. Sometimes he carries the exchange over into other social contexts as well. The example sounds trite: in everyday parlance, we might understand it as a way of 'getting a sense of what a guy is *really* like'. But his actions demonstrate a sophisticated appreciation of the performative agency of mediating environments. Identity is always relational and emerges through interaction: there is no underlying authentic self. Aware of how tightly framed and packaged digitally delivered sexual 'goods' tend to be, my informant counters this situation by embedding and 'migrating' the developing relationship across a range of different infrastructural environments. Like hookup apps, bars, restaurants and nightclubs are sociotechnical infrastructures that allow different attributes of a person or entity to emerge. Aware that different properties of a person emerge in different practical setups, this man's practice can be conceived as one that subjects the encounter to a series of multicontextual trials that might enable him to assess the potential multiplicity of whatever relational dynamic is coming to emerge between them.

In response to the instrumentality attributed to online dating sites, Badiou objects: 'nothing enables one to pre-arrange the encounter' (2012, p. 31). But there is another body of work in the French sociology of techniques that argues that passionate encounters *depend* on the sociomaterial arrangements and constraints in which they take place ('event-networks'). The experimental practice of making of new attachments is characterised here as a mix of preparative activities and passive surrender; the sort of receptivity that consists in *making oneself available* to transformation, to being 'swept aside', or newly affected (Gomart & Hennion 1999). When trying to think about what it might mean to plan or design queerer encounters, I came up with a fanciful idea that might multiply the 'pleasures of the unexpected' in digital worlds. Speculative designers describe their practice as 'a design process that disregards traditional utilitarian values in favour of playfulness, exploration and enjoyment . . . what is important is that [probes] provoke new design ideas and move both designers and participants out of their comfort zones' (Boehner, Gaver & Boucher 2012). Between speculating about speculative design and flicking between Badiou and Warner, I dreamt up an app that sets out playfully to disrupt our investments in pre-calculated desires; one that *glitches* and *misfires*, generating chance encounters in the vicinity of sex that neither party could precisely have intended. Some sort of cross between Grindr and Chatroulette[1] that incentivises the duration of the encounter (or 'gamifies' it) so that participants are persuaded to commit whatever time they can to find a way of relating that allows *something new to emerge*. And then just see what happens. It could be fun, or it could be a disaster. Who knows whether it will work, or what might be learned from it? But as Warner and Badiou demonstrate in their own distinctive ways, that is the scary and exciting thing about intimacy. It 'puts at risk the concrete world that is its given condition of possibility' (Warner 2002, p. 113).

'Call me maybe?'

As it turns out (and as is so often the case), just at the moment I was getting ready to pat myself on the back for inventing a widget with commercialisation potential (my University's Research Office would have been so pleased), I learned that popular culture had beaten me to the mark. Steve Kardynal, a YouTube celebrity who has made his name doing 'tragic' drag covers of various pop songs, has orchestrated a digital spectacle that teaches us a great deal about the queer potential of digital encounters. . . and uploaded it onto YouTube! In 'Call Me Maybe [Chatroulette version]', Kardynal lip-syncs along to Carly Rae Jepsen's 2012 pop hit of the same name, but every few instants gets paired with a new set of random strangers who become unwitting audients and respondents to his outlandish performances via the sorting and rotation functions of this digital platform (Kardynal 2012).

There is so much to love about this videoclip. Jepsen's upbeat paean to the spontaneous pleasures of hetero-feminine non-committal flirtation becomes a hyperbolic caricature of the instant gratification and seamless convenience promised by digital culture. Despite Badiou's self-professed penchant for random encounters with difference, I suspect Kardynal's exaggerated gender alterity would test even his limits (in fact, I'm quite sure of this). As the video proceeds, the viewer cannot help but become enwrapped in the multi-varied responses of the unsuspecting, randomised spectators to this outrageous effusion of queer silliness. It gradually becomes impossible to pull oneself away from the dynamic affective processes these strangers undergo as they flail around trying to find ways of relating to the queer spectacle that confronts them. From shock, disgust, boredom, horror and surprise to admiration, delight and shimmying amplifications of pleasure, these are mass subjects at their most becoming, caught in the very process of becoming-other. In sharing this video and making it available to the general public online, Kardynal enacts, amplifies and circulates precisely the queer delight in random encounters that I am investing here with speculative potential. What divine contagious affect (Gibbs 2001; Probyn 2005)!

When enjoying this cultural artefact, let us remind ourselves of how it does its work: Chatroulette serves here as a digital infrastructure that reduces the risks of danger, harm and reactionary violence sometimes associated with unexpected exposure to complete alterity (Race 2016). Much like the communal infrastructures of queer dance parties, which (as we saw in Chapter 2) invented new ways of reducing harm among their mass of excitable participants, and a little like the glory hole we encountered in Chapter 8, Chatroulette makes the most unlikely moments of interpersonal exchange and mutual enjoyment publicly available, all the while ensuring the relative safety of the direct participants in these encounters. In this sense, Kardynal's video might serve as a prototype for queer public health work today: it celebrates the generative pleasures of encounters across difference, while coming up with ways of ensuring these processes are safe enough to live with. The question becomes: what other infrastructures might we interfere with to foster such queer events? Which of them might be flexible enough and safe enough to play with? What needs to be perverted?

'It all depends on the chemistry'

On gay men's online profiles around the world, it is not unusual to find some version of the phrase 'it all depends on the chemistry' in the profile box where members are asked to specify what they are looking for. The phrase normally qualifies statements such as 'open to anything' – statements that are conspicuous for their steadfast rejection of the very terms of this prompt. Given the focus of the last two chapters, one could be forgiven that depending on the chemistry is veiled reference to chemsex. But that's not it – or at least, not in my experience. So what does this phrase mean? What strange chemistry is this? And what might it tell us about the queer potential of digital encounters?

'Chemistry' is the thing that the compatibility algorithms of commercial dating platforms promise to deliver but most often cannot. It references that special connection that is ever so hard to pin down but that makes a relationship durable enough to sustain the ongoing interest of participants while giving them occasions to differ. 'It all depends on chemistry' is distinctive in its refusal to specify the precise details of what it is looking for in advance. If the designs of digital sex tend to anticipate and suggest a user who knows what they want up front, the saying 'it all depends on the chemistry' is deliberately vague about the personal objectives or objectified attributes that motivate the desiring subject. In this sense, the statement resists the precalculative logic that digital devices try to configure in their users. Dodging the categories of prejudicial desire, it deploys the logic of the pharmakon to hold things open: 'let's take it as it comes'; 'let's see what happens'; 'why don't we let things eventuate and unfold?' Queer chemistry.

'It all depends on the chemistry' knows a thing or two about the contingencies of pleasure and its risks. If the erotic speculation undertaken on online hookup devices tends often to be populated according to fixed criteria, 'it all depends on chemistry' refuses the invitation to specify such selection criteria definitively in advance because it distrusts the efficacy of these devices to deliver what they claim but more importantly because it wants to take the risk of remaining open to the unknown possibilities of the encounter. These sexual alchemists are aware there is always the possibility of connections that overflow or exceed the fixtures of strict search criteria; that refusing such determinations might bring into play 'connections that we are in the habit of keeping separate' (Stengers 2015, p. 62); and that these connections brim with many more possibilities for textured pleasure, emergent intimacies and effective intervention into unwanted situations than any logic that 'ticks all the boxes' to stabilise desire, specify attributes and fix objects or identities is capable of delivering.

Framing, overflowing, eventuating, unfolding: these terms have been key to the argument of this book. Like queer traffic wardens, they try to keep open the intersection of sex and sociability by suspending the presumption that anyone entering this junction can know precisely in advance what circumstances they will encounter or what might emerge from it, however tightly it seems to be configured. These overflowing terms try to interrupt any precise predetermination of what might occasion risk and/or pleasure in a given situation, and in this sense they generate open futures – an altogether different relation to temporality and futurity than the dogmatic yes or no that queer optimists and pessimists quarrel over in relation to futures that they (or others) prescribe for us. Neither self-destructive hedonists nor redemptive pollyannas, I suspect that those who *attend to the chemistry* make the best friends and/or the most attentive, dynamic lovers. They know that pleasure and risk can eventuate in ways that overflow any initial framing or fixed prescription. Hit one of them up some time: oink, wink, woof – whatever it takes. Pay attention. See what happens: responsive attentiveness.

A gay science

If attending to the chemistry is a vernacular practice that gay men already put into practice, what sort of manner, what stance, what affective disposition should we adopt when attending to the unpredictable formulae of such chemistries? The gay science proposes an approach that affirms what is given in this world, and suggests that such an approach enables us to better grasp the possibilities of different situations in their contingency. Of what else would the gay science consist if not the affirmative possibility of working with contingencies? Contingency refers to the always provisional ways in which given entities touch, affect, colour, infuse, bleed into, infect each other – their knotty entanglements, the effects of which are entirely dependent on the manner in which they come together. As I have argued throughout, all relations are contingent, not just those between people. Working with contingencies involves careful experimentation with the nonhuman and human relations that constitute the infrastructure of our lives; infrastructures that provide the material support for our attachments, our practices, our pleasures, our ability to endure the world, and our sorrows; infrastructures that give shape to our movements, our feelings and our capacity to move on from situations. These infrastructures do more than mediate intimacy; they shape our capacities to endure the unsettling transformations that sex and intimacy and drug use often produce. The gay science proposes an affirmative art of attending to contingencies with a view to opening up possibilities in a manner that might just make a difference.

Some will say that it is easy for a white gay man to promote such a happy-go-lucky perspective on the contingencies of events. Others will worry: *contingencies are dangerous!* Events can be traumatic, if not monumentally disastrous. (Just look what happened in the USA in November 2016!) The election of the 45th US President is not an event any decent person could celebrate or really want to be a part of (*pace* Zizek). But become part of it we must, if we want actively to participate in the event's unfolding and change the meaning and identity of *'what just happened?!'* Moreover, affirming an event is not the same as celebrating it; to affirm something is to actively seize and grasp it in its present complexity – no cheerleading is necessary. How one proceeds from such an affirmation and translates it into a practical response is an ethical, situated and often critical challenge, and an open and active question.

It would be completely wrong to assume that gay men are unfettered by the determinations of gender, structural inequality, racial subordination, class, social disadvantage, etc. Compared to other subordinated groups, however, white gay men in Western countries have been subject to fewer soicomaterial determinations in recent history (especially since the introduction of effective antiretroviral therapy). Perhaps this is what has enabled many participants in gay culture to find ways of enjoying the contingent conditions of existence, comparatively unencumbered by sociomaterial determinisms and their dragging entanglements. But contingency has also been a source of precarity for homosexuals, faggots, clones, queers, sissies, poofters and trans-dudes, who have rarely benefited from, and still tend not to fare well against, the determined scripts of heteronormativity. For numerous queer, feminist and anti-racist critics, the most valiant or righteous way of countering these scripts, of chipping away at their onslaughts, is a stance of critical negativity – a stance that many have benefited from immeasurably. But in this book, I have chosen to follow another course, and explored the possibilities of cultivating an affirmative and positive perspective on the circumstances and conditions that mediate the possibilities of survival for a population disproportionately affected by HIV. There is so much one could get angry about, but I do not want to be an angry white man. Nor am I convinced that power is quite as monolithic as some proponents of queer negativity make out. Queer, inter-racial dance events are thriving in small pockets of urban and regional culture today despite the obstacles, while the bonds and allegiances of the social protest movements that are assembling in response to the present conjuncture are distinctive for how often they traverse established categories of identity. By their very existence, these examples (and there must be more) counter the presumption that white heteronormativity is all-determining. That is something I can work with. Indeed, it something that I *want* to work with. Gaily.

The affirmative approach to contingencies proposed in this book should not be taken as a prescription: gayness is certainly not the only way of handling indeterminacy and contingency. *How* we are affected by events, big and small, is one of the few choices we earthlings have, providing what little room we have for manoeuvre. There are many ways in which the unpredictability

of events might be approached, each with their consequences for the world and for what we might become. One all-too-common approach is to negate the possibilities generated by contingency, to try to eliminate or deny what is unfamiliar or doesn't conform to one's being as it is habitually enacted. But this strategy produces an entirely different subject than that anticipated by *The Gay Science*. A safer subject? Not necessarily, since the predilection to turn away from possibilities or refusal even to perceive them divests the perceiving subject of pragmatic capacities that are indispensable for responding to emergencies. An ignorant subject? Yes, if ignorance is merely taken to refer to the particular satisfaction that consists in ignoring certain possibilities. A conservative subject? No doubt, whether this quality is the upshot of having been hurt or burnt or timid or selfish or comfortable or lazy or privileged or just plain stubborn (people have their reasons). A fearful subject, to be sure: a cautious one at best. A Stoic subject, perhaps, but not all that pragmatic. It is hard to determine what the practice of denying or disavowing certain possibilities will produce: I will leave that experiment to others. But in any event, whatever subject emerges from these trials in self-mastery and control, I can tell you, it won't be a gay one.

Krishna in Erskinville

In the final stages of working on this book, Leon Fernandes, a young queer Indian-Australian artist and friend, launched an exhibition of his new work in a gallery attached to the Darlinghurst offices of a group of general practitioners who have served Sydney's HIV-positive and gay communities for over three decades. Leon's exhibition *Krishna in Erskinville* consists of several richly textured, colourfully woven artworks that depict Hindu deities in a range of mundane and everyday Australian suburban settings, and is the culmination of years of labour. Leon has kindly allowed me to reproduce an image of one of his pieces in this book (Figure 9.1). I cannot quite recall when or where I first met Leon – probably on some dance floor or other – but over the years I have become familiar with his contribution to counterpublic health, especially through his work for the NSW Users and AIDS Association.

Crafted with oils, spray paint, embroidery and cut-up remnants of neckties that once belonged to Leon's father, *Krishna in Erskinville* is a colourful, multi-layered work of entangled materials and queer hybridity. The work depicts the Hindu god of love, sex and beauty Krishna posing flirtatiously in front of the Imperial Hotel, an iconic Sydney queer neighbourhood pub, which also happens to be the birthplace of *Priscilla, Queen of the Desert* (Elliott 1994).[2] As the work's setting, the Imperial Hotel references the vibrant contribution that Australia's sexual subcultures have made to a creative cultural style that has become renowned internationally for its playful, irreverent, in-your-face creativity and colour (and is often taken to exhaust Australia's contribution to aesthetic innovation in popular culture completely). The name of the iconic hotel also references more obliquely the violent histories

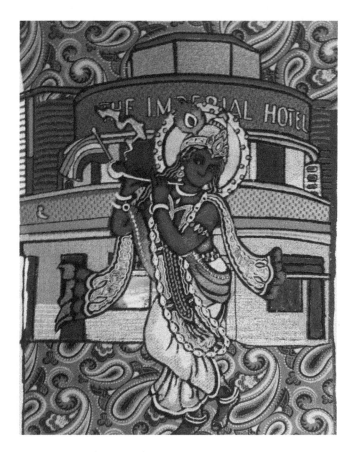

Figure 9.1 Krishna in Erskinville.

Artwork by Leon Fernandes, 2017. Courtesy of Leon Fernandes, photographed by Raf & Way Production, www.rafandway.com

of British imperialism, whose opportunistic and often violent exploitation of colonised lands and peoples has scarred not only the Indian subcontinent from which Leon's father hails, but also the original inhabitants of the Australian continent, the traditional owners of land stolen by white settlers to throw together the vitriolic mess now known as the Commonwealth of Australia – a remote outpost of 'splendid isolation', whose broken spirit and toxic public affects can be attributed largely to the nation's failure to acknowledge or address this violent, shameful historical legacy.

Fernandes' *Krishna* emerges from this complex, compromised, wild and violent landscape, festively adorned in peacock colours that echo the Gay Pride flag that flies off to the left. Krishna – who is also known as a lover, prankster, child and hero – stands precociously in front of this iconic gay pub brandishing a crystal pipe emanating a thick plume of intoxicating blue vapour, which rises languorously from the tip of the pipe. Fernandes is not heroicising or celebrating the meth user here; but nor is he denigrating or ridiculing this cheeky deity. The smoke of the pipe blends seamlessly into the built environment, and while the Gay Flag is flying, it functions as but one colourful addition to a landscape of vibrant conjoined fabrics and accoutrements that together constitute the joyous tapestry of this queer sub/urban aesthetic. Explaining his controversial decision to depict Krishna smoking crystal meth, Leon points to the ritual significance of drug consumption in many religions and communities around the world. But he also wants to make a concerted intervention into the contemporary materialisation of this substance within recent public culture: 'I wanted to lighten up the discourse around the "demon drug" and bring back a playful honesty about the various roles drugs play in our lives', he says. What better way to conclude *The Gay Science* than this surprising, life-affirming, joyous figuration of queer chemistry?

Fernandes understands that counterpublic health involves creative, multi-textured, collective contributions to the 'affective climates' of everyday life in which such disapproved, demonised and incriminating practices of consumption take place. Depicting an activity that, for many ordinary queer and other people, has become a mundane part of the pleasures and rhythms, ups and downs, highs and lows of everyday life, Fernandes is engaged in a perverse double manoeuvre in this work that seeks at once to affirm and deflate the drama surrounding 'the demon drug'. By playfully and directly foregrounding crystal meth as an unconcealed part of Australian queer life, *Krishna in Erskinville* produces this drug as a colourful, ancillary but otherwise unexceptional part of the rich urban fabric of life within Sydney's queer sexual subcultures and communities. In the process, he makes the drug available for more textured forms of attention and acknowledgement than the sensationalism that characterises the normative morality of the public sphere is able to deliver. The offending substance is imbued with a far more modulated and nuanced repertoire of affective responses than the *pleasing sort of terror* that normative publics want to make of it. Were a demon to steal into your loneliest loneliness, *Krisha in Erskinville* proposes new ways of hearing that demon out, replacing the melodramatic teeth-gnashing of Wagnerian triumphalism with a much more playful, friendly, unapologetic frankness that makes it possible to affirm what is given in this world, as it is lived now, in all its knotty but necessary contingency.

Notes

1 Chatroulette is an online website that pairs random users together for webcam-based conversations.
2 This movie, which features the travails of a group of drag queens on a road trip through the Simpson Desert, is renowned as Australia's first internationally famous queer blockbuster.

References

Ansell Pearson, K. 1997. *Viroid Life.* London: Routledge.

Arndt, J., Greenberg, J., Solomon, S., et al. 1997. Suppression, accessibility of death-related thoughts, and cultural worldview defense: Exploring the psychodynamics of terror management. *Journal of Personality & Social Psychology*, 73(1), pp. 5–18.

Badiou, A. 2012. *In Praise of Love.* London: Serpent's Tail.

Berlant, L. & Warner, M. 1998. Sex in public. *Critical Inquiry*, 24(2), pp. 547–566.

Boehner, K., Gaver, W. & Boucher, A. 2012. Probes. In C. Lury & N. Wakeford (eds.) *Inventive Methods: The Happening of the Social.* London: Routledge, pp. 185–201.

boyd, d. 2010. Social network sites as networked publics: Affordances, dynamics, and implications. In Z. Papacharissi (ed.) *A Networked Self: Identity, Community, and Culture on Social Network Sites.* New York: Routledge, pp. 39–58.

Callon, M. 1998. *The Laws of the Markets.* Oxford: Blackwell.

Dean, T. 2009. *Unlimited Intimacy.* Chicago: University of Chicago Press.

Elliott, S. 1994. *The Adventures of Priscilla, Queen of the Desert* [movie]. Universal City, CA: Gramercy Pictures.

Foucault, M. 2011. The gay science. *Critical Inquiry*, 37(3), pp. 385–403.

Gibbs, A. 2001. Contagious feelings: Pauline Hanson and the epidemiology of affect. *Australian Humanities Review*, 24, available at http://www.australianhumanities review.org/archive/Issue-December-2001/gibbs.html.

Goffman, E. 1963. *Stigma: Notes on the Management of Spoiled Identity.* London: Simon & Schuster Inc.

Gomart, E. & Hennion, A.1999. A sociology of attachment: Music amateurs, drug users. *The Sociological Review*, 47(S1), pp. 220–247.

Ito, M. 2008. Introduction. In K. Vernelis (ed.) *Networked Publics*. Cambridge, MA: MIT Press, pp. 1–14.

Kardynal, S. 2012. *Call me maybe – Chatroulette version.* Youtube.com [online]. Retrieved from https://www.youtube.com/watch?v=KAQhG59zqZc [28 February 2017].

Liu, P. 2015. *Queer Marxism in Two Chinas.* Durham: Duke University Press.

MacKee, F., 2016. Social media in gay London: Tinder as an alternative to hook-up apps. *Social Media+ Society*, 2(3), pp. 1–10.

Matsuda, M. 2005. Mobile communication and selective sociality. In M. Ito, D. Okabe & M. Matsuda (eds.) *Personal, Portable, Pedestrian: Mobile Phones in Japanese Life.* Cambridge, MA: MIT Press, pp. 123–142.

Payne, R. 2015. *The Promiscuity of Network Culture.* London: Routledge.

Probyn, E. 2005. *Blush: Faces of Shame.* Minneapolis: University of Minnesota Press.

Race, K. 2009. *Pleasure Consuming Medicine.* Durham: Duke University Press.

Race, K. 2016. The sexuality of the night: Violence and transformation. *Current Issues in Criminal Justice*, 28(1), pp. 105–110.

Stengers, I. 2015. *In Catastrophic Times.* London: Open Humanities Press.

Warner, M. 2002. *Publics and Counterpublics.* New York: Zone Books.

Index

For Product Safety Concerns and Information please contact our EU
representative GPSR@taylorandfrancis.com
Taylor & Francis Verlag GmbH, Kaufingerstraße 24, 80331 München, Germany